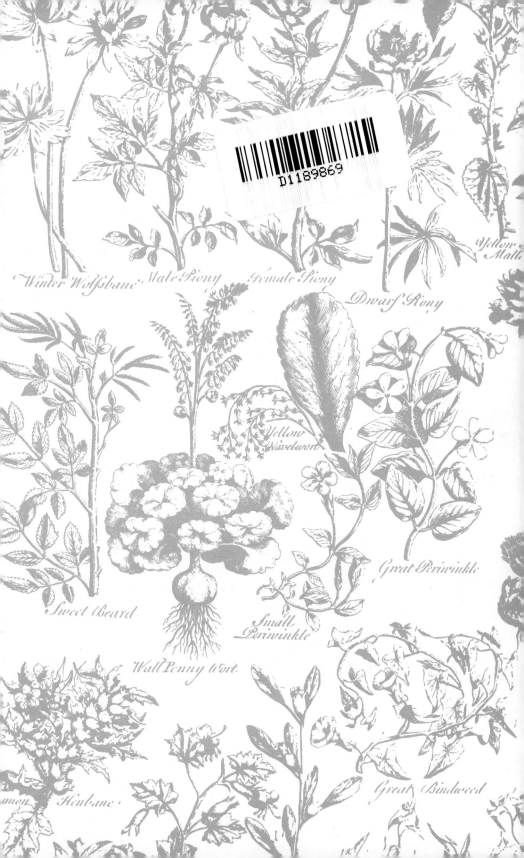

Winter Wolfsbane   Male Piony   Female Piony

Dwarf Piony

Yellow Malla

Yellow Navelwort

Great Periwinkle

Sweet Beard   Small Periwinkle

Wall Penny Wort

Henbane   Great Bindweed

PROVEN HERBAL REMEDIES

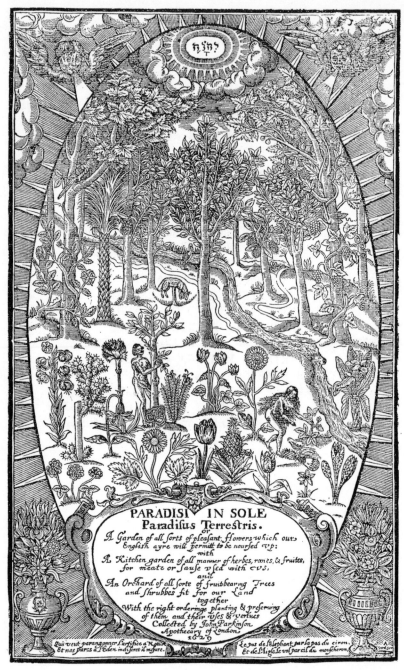

PARADISI IN SOLE
Paradisus Terrestris.
or
A Garden of all sorts of pleasant flowers which our
English ayre will permitt to be noursed vp:
with
A Kitchen garden of all manner of herbes, rootes, & fruites,
for meate or sause vsed with vs.
and
An Orchard of all sorte of fruitbearing Trees
and Shrubbes fit for our Land
together
With the right orderinge planting & preseruing
of them and their vses & vertues
Collected by John Parkinson
Apothecary of London.
1629

Qui veut parangonner l'artifice a Nature,
Et nos parcs à l'Eden. mal seret il mesure.

Le pas de l'elephant. par le pas du ciron,
Et de l'aigle le vol par cil du moucheron.

*From a volume in the collection of old and
modern herbals in the author's library.*

iv

PROVEN
HERBAL
REMEDIES

by John H. Tobe

With a section on
GENERAL RULES
for
GATHERING AND PRESERVING HERBS
By Thomas Green

PROVOKER PRESS
1969

v

Printed in Canada

DEDICATION

To all those men and women, wherever they are found on this earth, who believe in medical and healing freedom for all and who are willing to fight to the bitter end for this freedom, this volume is seriously dedicated.

It is my belief that no one should be forced to take or be injected with drugs of any kind; no one should be forced to undergo a blood transfusion, any more than anyone should be forced to undergo a heart or a kidney transplant operation.

I voice my profound admiration and respect for all those who have fought in the past and those who continue to fight so bravely in spite of continued persecution by over-zealous authorities.

APOLOGIA

It has been the general practice now for some years, when offering other means of healing than organized medicine, to give or state a disclaimer .... and the phrasing runs similar to this:

"The material, recipes, botanical materia medica compounds, infusions and decoctions in this book are not intended to replace the services of a physician or physicians. A physician should be consulted when the condition logically requires his services."

It has never been brought to my attention that such a statement or disclaimer is required or necessary by law. I would presume that this disclaimer was given to prevent legal action being taken against the author.

I hold no animosity towards the medical profession. In fact, I respect many members of this profession. But I do not in the slightest degree feel that they are the only, nor the best, nor the noblest profession in the healing arts.

I am not even slightly convinced that modern medicine, with the use of the thousands of synthetic drugs, has done one iota better in the treatment of disease than the herbalist and his herbs. In fact, it is absolutely true that while many or most drugs are harmful and create side effects ... which are often more serious than the disease being treated ... the herbalists do much better. I, for one, have never heard of a single instance of serious side effects from the use of prescribed herbs.

It is an acknowledged fact that a large percentage of all those hospitalized are there because of purely iatrogenic diseases.

Because I have seen so many members of various healing professions make the statement about consulting your doctor, I am led to believe that it is necessary for them to do so if they are to remain in practice. If this is compulsory according to the laws of the land, I of course, will have no alternative but to comply, and this article is, in fact, my complaisance.

However, to the best of my knowledge, we still have freedom of the press in Canada and I boldly state that every human being holds an inherent right to select the method of healing or the healer of his choice.

I do not suggest that herbs are the only or even the best form of healing, but I do emphatically claim that herbalism is mankind's oldest form of healing.

I further maintain that each individual has the right to read, to study, to investigate and then decide on the method or kind of healing that he thinks is best suited to his needs.

Forthrightly I state, if your condition requires the attention of a surgeon, then of course that is where you should go for assistance. If you feel that the removal of a gland, a protuberance, an organ or any other part of your anatomy is necessary for your well-being, then of course the logical choice is a surgeon. If you feel that you desire to be inoculated, vaccinated, injected or treated by a medical practitioner, then by all means that is where you should go.

By the same token, if you believe that a chiropractor, an osteopath, a podiatrist, a naturopath, a spiritual healer, a fasting specialist, a psychiatrist or a herbalist will best fulfill your needs, then of course it should be your right or privilege to consult him.

It is not my intent at this time to enter into a discussion concerning the merits, the qualifications or the implications involved in comparing the various schools of healing. I simply categorically contend that each individual has the right to choose his mode or method of healing.

TABLE OF CONTENTS

COMPREHENSIVE ALPHABETICAL LIST OF AILMENTS

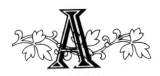

ACNE AND OTHER SKIN AFFECTIONS

PLANT: Fumitory   *Fumaria officinalis*
WHERE FOUND: Europe and Asia
PART USED: Herb
ACTION: Aperient, diuretic, slightly tonic
DISSERTATION: Used mainly in stomach disorders and skin affections.

Gerard writes: "Dioscorides affirmeth that the juice of Fumitory, of that which groweth among Barley, with gum Arabic, doth take away unprofitable hairs that prick the eyes, growing upon the eye lids, the hairs that prick first plucked away, for it will not suffer others to grow in their place."

Culpeper writes: "The juice of the Fumitory and Docks mingled with vinegar and the places gently washed therewith, cures all sorts of scabs, pimples, blotches, wheals and pushes which arise on the face or hands or any other part of the body."

METHOD: Infusion of 1 oz. to 1 pt. of boiling water
DOSAGE: Wineglassful every 3 hours

> John Hill, M.D. (1756) says: "Some smoke the dried leaves in the manner of tobacco for disorders of the head with success."

ACUTE MANIA — MUSCULAR TWITCHING

PLANT: Hemlock   *Conium maculatum*
WHERE FOUND: Europe and Great Britain
PART USED: Leaves and unripe fruits
ACTION: Anodyne, sedative
DISSERTATION: Recognized of particular service in all spasmodic affections; e.g., chorea, acute mania and epilepsy. Good for whooping cough.

> NOTE: An overdose can produce paralysis. Extremely dangerous and must be administered only by a qualified practitioner.

In the above the Hebrew word is rendered as 'Gall' and it seems certain that it refers to Hemlock. It is known that Hemlock was used in ancient days to put criminals to death, and others suffered the same fate who would not today be classed as criminals. It will be remembered that Socrates drank a draught of Hemlock juice. The Jews in ancient days used Hemlock to deaden the pains of dying criminals. Such as were being stoned to death were frequently given a cup of wine containing myrrh and Hemlock juice to deaden their death pains. It is thought that as Jesus hung upon the cross he was given vinegar, myrrh and Hemlock.
METHOD: From leaves, powdered leaves. From seeds, liquid extract.
DOSAGE: Powdered leaves, 2-8 gr.; Liquid extract, 2-5 min.

ACUTE TONSILITIS

PLANT: Hellebore, American   *Veratrum viride*
WHERE FOUND: Canada and the United States
PART USED: Rhizome

ACTION: Cardiac depressant
DISSERTATION: An excellent remedy for acute tonsilitis, and as a gargle for sore throat. Most useful in febrile and inflammatory affection of the respiratory organs. Relieves irritation of the nervous system and is highly regarded as a remedy in convulsions, mania, neuralgia and headache. It is a known poison and should be used with care and caution.
METHOD: Powdered root
DOSAGE: 1 to 2 gr.

AFFECTIONS OF THE GUMS

PLANT: Columbine, Common   *Aquilegia vulgaris*
WHERE FOUND: Southern France
PART USED: Seeds
ACTION: Antiphlogistic
DISSERTATION: In Thomas Green's 'Universal Herbal' we read: "Hill observes, that the seeds operate by sweat and urine, open obstructions of the viscera, and are good in the jaundice, in fevers, and in the smallpox and measles, to throw out the pustules. A decoction of the leaves is good for sore throats, and a tincture of the flowers in brandy is recommended by Tournefort as an excellent gargle for scorbutic affections of the gums."

"Culpeper informs us, that the Spaniards eat a piece of the root in a morning fasting, many days together, when troubled with the stone."

3

AFFECTIONS OF THE URINARY PASSAGES

PLANT: St. Johns Wort   *Hypericum perforatum*
WHERE FOUND: Europe
PART USED: Herb
ACTION: Astringent, diuretic, expectorant
DISSERTATION: It is highly esteemed in affections of the urinary passages.
METHOD: Infusion of 1 oz. herb to 1 pt. boiling water
DOSAGE: Wineglassful doses

AGUE

PLANT: Calamus   *Acorus calamus*
WHERE FOUND: Throughout Europe and Britain
PART USED: Rhizome
ACTION: Aromatic, carminative, stomachic
DISSERTATION: Useful in flatulence, wind, colic, ague. An old remedy for ague. This root was known to the ancient Greek and Arabian doctors. The fresh candied root was used by the Indians and the Turks for dyspepsia.
METHOD: Infusion of 1 oz. to 1 pt. boiling water
DOSAGE: Taken freely in teacupful doses

ALCOHOLISM

PLANT: Gold Thread   *Coptis trifolia*
WHERE FOUND: India. However the variety *groelandica*, which is equal in medicinal value, grows in Canada and the United States.
PART USED: Rhizome

ACTION: A decoction of Gold Thread will frequently destroy the desire for alcoholic beverages. A bitter tonic.

DISSERTATION: Its excellent qualities should be better known. It improves the appetite, promotes digestion and acts as a general stimulant to the system. Highly beneficial in convalescence. Has been proven useful in chronic inflammation of the stomach. Soothes irritation of the mouth.

METHOD: Steep a teaspoonful of the powdered root in a cup of boiling water

DOSAGE: Teaspoonful 4 or 5 times daily

AMAUROSIS
(Loss of Vision without Pathological Indications)

PLANT: Arnica   *Arnica montana*

WHERE FOUND: Europe

PART USED: Rhizome, flowers, leaves

ACTION: Diaphoretic, diuretic, emmenagogue, stimulant, sudorific, vulnerary

DISSERTATION: In "Materia Medica Vegetabilis" written by E. F. Steinmetz, we read: "The flowers in the form of a tincture work on the circulation organs, particularly on the capillary vessels, secondary also on the respiration organs. The circulation of the blood is accelerated, the frequency of the pulse and the respiration and the secretion of sweat are considerably increased. A further application of Arnica is in cases of spinal paralysis and concussion of the brain, and atonic diarrhoea. The haemostatic action in cases of external and also of internal bleedings is well known. The flowers made into an electuary with honey, have the reputation of curing intermittent fevers."

"Arnica leaves. They are used in fever, against paralysis and as a vulnerary. They act as a strong sternutatory."

"Arnica root. It is used chiefly in the form of tincture as

5

a popular application to bruises and chilblains; internally it is prescribed as a stimulant and sudorific."

In Matthew Robinson's herbal we read: "The plant possesses very great virtues... It is given in amaurosis, paralysis, and other nervous affections. It has been recommended for hydrocephalous, and typhous fevers, especially in the latter stages."

Haller says, "that even gutta serena, or loss of sight, has yielded to the powers of this medicine."

Robinson goes on to say, "It is also recommended in chronic rheumatism; in retention of the urine, from paralysis of the bladder; in intermittent fevers, when combined with Peruvian bark, where it has been very efficacious; in putrid diseases; to promote the uterine discharge; and in internal pains and congestions, from bruises.

"The flowers," say an eminent physician, "are stimulating and discutient. In small doses, and properly administered, they produce very beneficial effects, in raising the pulse, in exciting the action of the whole sanguinerous system, in checking diarrhoeas, in promoting expectoration, and especially in removing paralytic affections of the voluntary muscles; but they are frequently attended with no sensible operation, except that in some cases of paralysis, the cure is said to be preceded by a peculiar pricking, and by shooting pains in the affected parts."

ANAEMIA

PLANT: Cicely, Sweet   *Myrrhis odorata*
WHERE FOUND: Common British and European plant
PART USED: Herb, root
ACTION: Carminative, expectorant, stomachic
DISSERTATION: The fresh root eaten freely has proven useful for coughs and flatulence, as well as a gentle stimulant in indigestion and stomachic disorders. The dried root is best made into a decoction and the herb is best made into an infusion. An infusion made from the herb gives good results for anaemia, and is a splendid tonic for young girls.
METHOD: Decoction of 1 oz. root to 1 pt. boiling water; infusion of 1 oz. herb to 1 pt. boiling water

ANGINA PECTORIS

PLANT: Mescal Buttons or Pellote   *Lopophora lewinii*
WHERE FOUND: North Mexico and Texas
PART USED: Fruit. The sacred mushroom of the Aztecs
ACTION: Cardiac, emetic, narcotic, tonic
DISSERTATION: Remember, this is a narcotic and has a reputation in angina pectoris, paroxysmal complaints and dyspnoea. This drug has to be treated with caution, for it causes emises even when taken in small quantities.

ANTIDOTE TO POISONS - BALDNESS

PLANT: Southernwood or Old Man   *Artemisia abrotanum*
WHERE FOUND: Europe, and also widely grown garden plant
PART USED: Herb
ACTION: Antiseptic, detergent, emmenogogue, stimulant
DISSERTATION: It is recommended by the old herbalists as an

antidote to poisons and it was said that the burnt herb would drive away serpents.
METHOD: Liquid extract
DOSAGE: ½ - 1 dr.

Culpeper writes, "The ashes thereof dries up and heals old ulcers that are without inflammation ... The ashes mixed with old salad oil helps those that have hair fallen and are bald, causing the hair to grow again either on the head or beard."

ANTISPASMODIC

PLANT: Cedron   *Simaba cedron*
WHERE FOUND: Central America
PART USED: Seeds
ACTION: Antispasmodic, bitter, fever reducer, sedative, tonic
DISSERTATION: The exceedingly bitter seeds have been used in malarial complaints, dyspepsia and intermittent fevers.
METHOD: Infusion of 1 oz. to 1 pt. boiling water
DOSAGE: 1 tablespoonful 3 or 4 times a day

APHRODISIAC

PLANT: Damiana   *Turnera diffusa*
WHERE FOUND: Sub-tropical America, Africa and Texas
PART USED: Leaves
ACTION: Aphrodisiac, diuretic, tonic

DISSERTATION: Damiana is very largely prescribed on account of its aphrodisiac qualities, and there is no doubt that it has a very great general and beneficial action on the reproductive organs. It also acts as a tonic to the nervous system.
METHOD: Extract of Damian
DOSAGE: 5 to 10 gr.

APHRODISIAC

PLANT: Celery   *Apium graveolens*
WHERE FOUND: Southern Europe, but widely grown as a vegetable
PART USED: Seeds and stalks
ACTION: Aphrodisiac, carminative, diuretic, tonic
DISSERTATION: It is recommended in rheumatism and arthritis. Culpeper advised the use of the seeds, plant and roots for various complaints.
METHOD: Liquid extract
DOSAGE: 5 to 20 min.

ARTHRITIS AND MALNUTRITION

PLANT: Lucerne or Alfalfa   *Medicago sativa*
WHERE FOUND: Europe and America; wherever cattle are raised
PART USED: Whole herb
ACTION: Alterative, nutritive
DISSERTATION: Known generally as alfalfa. It is known best as one of the finest of all grasses for cattle. Its nutritive value has been recognized for centuries. Widely used for arthritis,

where the powdered herb is taken with cider vinegar and honey: one teaspoonful of each in a glass of water. Has long been used as a strengthening and weight adding tonic.

> Dioscorides back in the first century prescribed a concoction that he called 'OXYMEL' for the treatment of arthritis, epilepsy and snake-bite. 'OXYMEL' literally translated means sour honey, and the first English translator wrote it as Vinegar-Honey.

ARTICULAR STIFFNESS

PLANT: Poison Oak   *Rhus toxicodendron*
WHERE FOUND: North America
PART USED: Leaves
ACTION: Irritant, narcotic, stimulant
DISSERTATION: Valuable in articular stiffness and acute rheumatism. Also has been used with success in the treatment of obstinate skin diseases and in small doses is an excellent sedative for the nervous system.
METHOD: Liquid extract
DOSAGE: 5 to 30 drops

ASTHMA

PLANT: Butterbur   *Petasites vulgaris*
WHERE FOUND: Europe and North Asia

PART USED: Root
ACTION: Cardiac, diuretic, stimulant, tonic
DISSERTATION: Has long been in use as a remedy in fevers, asthma, colds and urinary complaints, gravel and plague. A stimulant for weak heart and good in dropsy.
METHOD: Decoction of 1 oz. in 1 pt. boiling water
DOSAGE: Frequent wineglassful doses

ATROPHY OF TESTES AND MAMMAE

PLANT: Saw Palmetto   *Serenoa serrulata*
WHERE FOUND: Eastern North America
PART USED: Berry
ACTION: Diuretic, nutritive, sedative, tonic
DISSERTATION: Has a marked effect on all the glandular tissues for it builds up strength and flesh rapidly. Should be used in atrophy of testes and mammae.
METHOD: Powdered berries
DOSAGE: 15 gr.

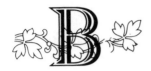

BARRENNESS AND PAIN RELIEVER

PLANT: Catnep   *Nepeta cataria*
WHERE FOUND: Native to England but found in North America
PART USED: Herb
ACTION: Carminative, diaphoretic, refrigerant, tonic
DISSERTATION: Produces free perspiration, useful in colds, also relieves pains and flatulence.

Catnep gets its name from the liking of cats for this plant. It is said that when it starts to wither they will roll themselves in it and chew it. There is an old belief that it makes cats 'frolicsome, amorous and full of battle.'
METHOD: Infusion of 1 oz. to 1 pt. boiling water
DOSAGE: For children: 2 or 3 teaspoonfuls; Adults: 2 tablespoonfuls

---

There is also an ancient saying that "if the root be chewed it will make the most quiet person fierce and quarrelsome."

BEAUTIFYING AGENT

PLANT: Frostwort or Rock Rose   *Helianthemum canadense*
WHERE FOUND: Europe, Great Britain and America
PART USED: Herb
ACTION: Alterative, astringent, tonic
DISSERTATION: Taken internally as a remedy for scrofula. Used externally as a wash for ulcers and sores.

Gerard writes: "Pliny writeth the Helianthemum grows ... in the mountains of Cicilia near the sea; saying further, that the wise men of these countries and the Kings of Persia do anoint their bodies herewith, boiled with Lion's fat, a little Saffron and Wine of Dates, that they may seem fair and beautiful ..."
METHOD: Infusion of 1 oz. to 1 pt. boiling water
DOSAGE: Wineglassful doses taken freely

BELLY OPENER

PLANT: All-Heal or Wound-Wort   *Brunella vulgaris*
WHERE FOUND: Europe
PART USED: Herb
ACTION: Antiseptic, antispasmodic
DISSERTATION: In Culpeper's herbal we read: "It kills the worms, helps the gout, cramps, and convulsions; provokes urine, and helps all joint aches. It helps all cold griefs of the head, the vertigo, falling sickness, the lethargy, the wind colic, obstructions of the liver and spleen, stone in the kidneys and bladder. It provokes the terms, expels the dead birth: it is excellent for the griefs of the sinews, itch, stone, and toothache, the bite of mad dogs and venomous beasts, and purgeth choler very gently."
METHOD: Bruised leaves are applied to wounds. Fresh juice is

14

made into a syrup

DOSAGE: Syrup made from fresh juice is taken internally a teaspoonful at a time

BELLYACHE OR PAINS OF COLIC

PLANT: Mullein   *Verbascum thapsus*

WHERE FOUND: Well known garden plant; native to the Mediterranean area

PART USED: Leaves and flowers

ACTION: Astringent, demulcent, pectoral

DISSERTATION: Gerard states: "The leaves are worn under the feet in a manner of a shoe sole or sock and assist to bring down in young maidens their desired sickness being so kept under their feet that they do not fall away." And also: "The later physicians commend the yellow flowers being steeped in oil and set in warm dung until they be washed into the oil and consumed away, to be a remedy for piles."

Culpeper writes: "A decoction of the leaves thereof and of Sage, Marjoram and Camomile Flowers and the places bathed therewith, that have the sinews stiff with cold or cramp doth bring them much ease and comfort . . ." "The juice of the leaves and flowers being laid upon rough warts, and also the powder of the dried roots rubbed on, doth easily take them away, but doth no good to smooth warts . . . The powder of the dried flowers is an especial remedy for those that are troubled with the belly-ache or the pains of colic."

BILIARY CONCRETIONS

PLANT: Olive   *Olea europaea*
WHERE FOUND: Mediterranean lands
PART USED: Oil
ACTION: Aperient, emolient, nutritive
DISSERTATION: Through the ages it has been used internally as a remedy for bowel diseases, habitual constipation, lead colic, for removing worms and in large doses dispels biliary concretions. Externally it forms an important role in embrocations, ointments and liniments, used in bruises, burns, scalds, rheumatic and skin ailments. Proven valuable as an inunction for teething children, keeping the bowels regular and acting as a tonic by absorption.
METHOD: The best virgin oil should be obtained
DOSAGE: From a teaspoonful to 2 tablespoonfuls as indicated

BINDINGS

PLANT: Bilberry   *Vaccinium myrtilllus*
WHERE FOUND: On the heaths in Great Britain
PART USED: Ripe fruits and leaves
ACTION: Astringent, diuretic, refrigerant
DISSERTATION: Culpeper says "They are under the dominion of Jupiter. It is a pity they are used no more in physic than they are. The black bilberries are good in hot agues, and to cool the heat of the liver and stomach: they do somewhat bind the belly, and stay the vomitings and loathings: the juice of the berries made into a syrup, or the pulp made into a conserve with sugar, is good for the purposes aforesaid, as also for an old cough, or an ulcer in the lungs, or other diseases therein. The red whorts are more binding, and stop women's courses, spitting of blood or any other flux of blood or humours, being used as

16

well outwardly as inwardly."
METHOD: 1 teaspoon of berries or leaves to a cup of boiling water
DOSAGE: Take 1 to 2 cupfuls during the day in mouthful doses

A combination of thyme, strawberry and bilberry leaves make a delightful nutritive tea.

BITE OF MAD DOGS

PLANT: Horehound, Black   *Ballota nigra*
WHERE FOUND: Europe
PART USED: Herb
ACTION: Antispasmodic, stimulant, vermifuge
DISSERTATION: The herb is used very little in modern botanical medicine although the ancients continuously extolled its worth.

Dioscorides says: "The leaves beaten with salt and applied to the wound cure the bite of mad dogs."

BITES OF VENOMOUS BEASTS

PLANT: Bugloss   *Echium vulgare*

17

WHERE FOUND: Canary Islands, Madeira and West Asia
PART USED: Herb
ACTION: Demulcent, diuretic, expectorant
DISSERTATION: Gerard writes: "The herb chewed and the juice swallowed down is a most singular remedy against poison and the biting of any venomous beast; and the root so chewed and laid upon the sore works the same effect."
METHOD: Infusion of 1 oz. to 1 pt. boiling water
DOSAGE: Wineglassful to teacupful doses as required

> Dioscorides says that, if the leaves be held in the hand, no venomous creatures will come near the holder to sting him for that day.

BLACK AND BLUE MARKS ON SKIN

PLANT: Bay Tree   *Laurus nobilis*
WHERE FOUND: Europe
PART USED: Leaves, fruits, oil
ACTION: Stomachic
DISSERTATION: In Culpeper's Herbal we read: "Galen said, that the leaves or bark do dry and heal very much, and the berries more than the leaves; the bark of the root is less sharp and hot, but more bitter, and hath some astrictions withal, whereby it is effectual to break the stone, and good to open obstructions of the liver, spleen, and other inward parts which bring the jaundice, dropsy, etc. ... The oil takes away the marks of the skin and flesh by bruises, falls, etc. and dissolveth the congealed blood in them. It helpeth also the itch, scabs, and

weals in the skin."

BLADDER, GRAVEL AND KIDNEY COMPLAINTS

PLANT: Parsley Piert   *Alchemilla arvensis*
WHERE FOUND: Europe
PART USED: Herb
ACTION: Demulcent, diuretic
DISSERTATION: Long used in cases of gravel, kidney and bladder complaints. It acts directly on the parts affected, and will be found exceedingly valuable even in seemingly incurable cases. Several London doctors prescribe this remedy regularly.
    Although John Miller says "the vulgar have a great opinion of it" and "it is seldom prescribed by physicians" yet it was a herb known to the ancients and spoken of highly by Gerard and Culpeper.
METHOD: Infusion of 1 oz. herb to 1 pt. boiling water
DOSAGE: Teacupful doses three times a day

BLEEDING, TO STOP

PLANT: Love-Lies-Bleeding   *Amaranthus hypochondriacus*
WHERE FOUND: Native to Persia but widely cultivated everywhere
PART USED: Flowers and plant
ACTION: Astringent, corrective, haemostatic
DISSERTATION: It is used externally as an application in ulcerated conditions; as a douche in leucorrhoea; and as a wash for ulcers.
    Culpeper writes: "The flowers dried and beaten into powder, stop the terms in women, and so do almost all other

red things. And by the icon or image of every herb, the ancients at first found out their virtues. Modern writers laugh at them for it; but I wonder in my heart how the virtue of herbs came at first to be known, if not by their signatures; the moderns have them from the writings of the ancients; the ancients had no writings to have them from: but to proceed — The flowers stop all fluxes of blood, whether in man or woman, bleeding either at the nose or wound."
METHOD: Decoction
DOSAGE: Wineglassful doses as needed

BLEEDING OF THE LUNGS

PLANT: Liverwort, American   *Anemone hepatica*
WHERE FOUND: North America
PART USED: Herb
ACTION: Astringent, pectoral, tonic
DISSERTATION: Because of the pectoral qualities it may be used for bleeding of the lungs, chest conditions and coughs. Also, a mild remedy in disorders of the liver and indigestion.
METHOD: Infusion of 1 oz. herb to 1 pt. boiling water
DOSAGE: ½ teacupful frequently

BLEEDING OF MINOR WOUNDS

PLANT: Plantain   *Plantago major*
WHERE FOUND: Common weed almost everywhere
PART USED: Leaves
ACTION: Alterative, cooling, diuretic
DISSERTATION: The fresh leaves will stay bleeding of minor wounds. When the fresh leaves are rubbed on parts of the body

stung by insects or nettles, they will act as a cool and give relief.
METHOD: Infusion of 1 oz. leaves to 1 pt. boiling water
DOSAGE: Wineglassful doses

BLIND STAGGERS (Meagrims)

PLANT: Tansy, Common   *Tannacetum vulgare*
WHERE FOUND: Europe
PART USED: Leaves
ACTION: Anthelmintic, emmenagogue, resolvent, stomachic, tonic
DISSERTATION: Culpeper says it is "good to stop all kinds of fluxes and preternatural evacuations, to dissolve congealed blood, to help those who are bruised by falls: outwardly it is used as a cosmetic, to take off freckles, sunburn and morphew; as also in restrigent gargarisms."
METHOD: 1 oz. to 1 pt. boiling water
DOSAGE: Taken in teacupful doses morning and night

BLISTERED SURFACES

PLANT: Mezereon   *Daphne mezereum*
WHERE FOUND: Native to the mountainous areas of Europe; cultivated in Great Britain
PART USED: Bark, root, root-bark
ACTION: Alterative, diuretic, stimulant
DISSERTATION: Externally it is used as a lotion for blistered surfaces and indolent ulcers. Acts favorably in scrofula and rheumatism when taken internally.
METHOD: Decoction of ½ oz. powdered root-bark in 1 pt. of water
DOSAGE: Wineglassful doses

BLOOD IMPURITIES AND BURNS

PLANT: Burdock   *Arctium lappa*
WHERE FOUND: Europe
PART USED: Root, herb, fruit and seeds
ACTION: Alterative, diaphoretic, diuretic
DISSERTATION: Considered the finest blood purifier in the botanical kingdom.

     John Parkinson states, "The juice of the leaves given to drink with old wine doth wonderfully help the bitings of any serpents, as also of the mad dog."
METHOD: Root and seed, either or both, taken as a decoction: 1 oz. to 1½ pts. of water, boiled down to 1 pt.
DOSAGE: Wineglassful 3 or 4 times a day

     Also, "The leaves being bruised with the white of an egg and laid on any place burnt with fire doth take out the fire, giveth sudden ease and heals it up afterwards."

BLOOD IMPURITIES AND SCURVY

PLANT: Brooklime   *Veronica beccabunga*
WHERE FOUND: Throughout Europe, almost always near water and frequently in beds of watercress
PART USED: Herb

ACTION: Alterative, antiscorbutic, antiscrofulous, diuretic
DISSERTATION: It is given in scurvy and impurities of the blood. Also claimed to have the ability to pulverize bladder stone and pass the gravel away.
METHOD: Infusion of 1 oz. of leaves to 1 pt. boiling water
DOSAGE: Frequent wineglassful doses

BODY HEAT GENERATOR — COLDNESS OF EXTREMITIES

PLANT: Bayberry   *Myrica cerifera*
WHERE FOUND: Widely distributed in America and Eurasia
PART USED: Bark
ACTION: Astringent, stimulant, tonic
DISSERTATION: Said to be one of the most useful and beneficial herbs in botanic medicure. Forms the basis of the celebrated composition powder.
METHOD: 1 oz. powdered bark to 1 pt. boiling water
DOSAGE: Drink when warm, as tea

BRIGHT'S DISEASE

PLANT: Button Snakeroot   *Liatris spicata*
WHERE FOUND: North America
PART USED: Rhizome
ACTION: Diuretic, stimulant
DISSERTATION: It acts kindly on the stomach and is of value in kidney diseases. Said to be beneficial in Bright's disease. Has also been used effectively in the treatment of gonorrhoea.
METHOD: Infusion of 1 oz. to 1 pt. water
DOSAGE: Wineglassful doses 3 or 4 times a day

BRONCHIAL, LARYNGEAL, PULMONARY AFFECTIONS

PLANT: Sunflower   *Helianthus annuus*
WHERE FOUND: America, Europe, Asia
PART USED: Seeds, leaves
ACTION: Diuretic, expectorant
DISSERTATION: For years this plant has been used in bronchial, laryngeal and pulmonary affections, coughs and colds.
METHOD: 2 oz. Sunflower seeds and 1 qt. water boiled down to 12 oz. and strained. Add 6 oz. Hollands gin and 6 oz. sugar.
DOSAGE: 1 to 2 teaspoonfuls frequently during the day

BRONCHITIS, BRONCHIAL PNEUMONIA AND PHTHISIS

PLANT: Cocillana   *Guarea rusbyi*
WHERE FOUND: South America, the eastern Andes
PART USED: Bark
ACTION: Expectorant
DISSERTATION: Small doses act as an expectorant; large doses are emetic in action.
METHOD: Powdered bark
DOSAGE: 8 to 15 gr.

BROKEN BONES

PLANT: Solomon's Seal   *Polygonatum multiflorum*
WHERE FOUND: Native to North America
PART USED: Rhizome
ACTION: Astringent, demulcent, tonic
DISSERTATION: Gerard writes: "Galen saith that neither herb

nor root thereof is to be given inwardly; but not what experience hath found out specially among the vulgar sort of people in Hampshire which Galen, Dioscorides or any other that have written about plants have not so much as dreamed of; which is that if any of what age or sex soever chance to have any bones broken in what part of their bodies soever their refuge is to stamp the root hereof and give it unto the patient in ale to drink, which sodereth and glues together the bones in very short space and very strongly, yea though the bones be but slenderly and unhandsomely placed and wrapped up . . ."

> "Matthiolas teacheth that the water is drawn out of the roots wherewith the women of Italy use to scoure their faces from sunne-browning, freckles, morphew or any such deformities of the skin."

BRUISES AND SWELLINGS

PLANT: Arnica   *Arnica montana*
WHERE FOUND: Northern hemisphere
PART USED: Rhizome, flowers
ACTION: Stimulant, vulnerary
DISSERTATION: This plant is one of the most widely used herbs in homeopathy, for varied conditions including neuralgic pains, pains caused by overstrain of muscles, sinews and joints, spinal paralysis, intermittent fever, concussion, chilblains, bruises and swellings.
METHOD:**Do not use internally as it is poisonous.** Use only as a local application.

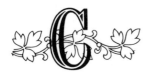

CARDIAC CONDITIONS

PLANT: Foxglove   *Digitalis purpurea*
WHERE FOUND: Europe and Great Britain, but grown everywhere in gardens
PART USED: Leaves
ACTION: Cardiac tonic, diuretic, sedative
DISSERTATION: Digitalis is a poisonous plant and should be used with care and under proper supervision. Used in cardiac complaints arising from kidney diseases; also in dropsy and urinary suppression. Known to have cumulative action.

Gerard says: "The Fox-gloves, in that they are bitter, are hot and dry, with a certain kind of cleansing quality joined therewith; yet they are of no use, neither have they any place amongst medicines, according to the Ancients."
METHOD: Infusion of 1 dr. in 1 pt. boiling water
DOSAGE: Teaspoonful doses only as directed

CATARACT, LENTICULAR AND CAPSULAR

PLANT: Cineraria Maritima   *Senecio maritimus*
WHERE FOUND: Native to West Indies, but introduced into most countries. Plants are readily available and are called Dusty

27

Miller.
PART USED: Juice of the plant
ACTION: Unknown
DISSERTATION: A trial is suggested before resorting to surgery.
METHOD: Expressed juice of plant is sterilized
DOSAGE: Applied to the eye with an eye dropper

CATARRH

PLANT: Benne   *Sesamum indicum*
WHERE FOUND: Native to India; cultivated in warm climates
PART USED: Leaves
ACTION: Demulcent, laxative
DISSERTATION: The fresh leaves are used in catarrhal affections, diarrhoea, dysentery, affections of kidney and bladder. The native Indians steep a few leaves in water and drink the mucilaginous juice freely. Externally they use it for eye inflammation and skin complaints.
METHOD: The natives steep a few leaves in water
DOSAGE: Drink freely

CHAPPED HANDS

PLANT: Sanicle   *Sanicula europaea*
WHERE FOUND: Europe
PART USED: Herb
ACTION: Astringent, alterative
DISSERTATION: Culpeper says this plant will cure "the wounds and mischiefs Mars inflicts upon the body of man."
John Miller describes it as one of the primary vulnerary

plants.

> Parkinson writes: "The country people who live where it groweth do use it to anoint their hands when they are chapt by the wind..."

CHEST, LUNG, STOMACH AND KIDNEY COMPLAINTS

PLANT: Balm of Gilead   *Populus candicans*
WHERE FOUND: Arabia
PART USED: Buds
ACTION: Diuretic, stimulant, sudorific, tonic
DISSERTATION: This plant has been highly rated since time immemorial. The buds are used in making an ointment used for all sorts of wounds, scalds, gout, piles and to promote growth of hair. It has been used against gout, rheumatism, bronchitis, intermittent fever and sciatics. Balsamic odour and bitter taste.
METHOD: As an ointment massaged into the affected parts

CHILDREN'S DIARRHOEA

PLANT: Meadowsweet   *Spiraea ulmaria*
WHERE FOUND: Found in the meadows and woods of Great Britain and Europe
PART USED: Herb
ACTION: Aromatic, astringent, diuretic
DISSERTATION: Pleasant to the taste and widely used in herb

beers. Good remedy in strangury, dropsy and children's diarrhoea, for which it is deemed a specific.
METHOD: Infusion of 1 oz. herb to 1 pt. boiling water
DOSAGE: Wineglassful doses as called for

Parkinson writes: "... many doe much delight therein to have it laid in their chambers, parlors, etc., and Queen Elizabeth of famous memory, did more desire it than any other sweet herb to strew her chambers withall ..."

CHRONIC AFFECTIONS OF THE MUCOUS AIR PASSAGES

PLANT: Galbanum *Ferula galbaniflua*
WHERE FOUND: Persia and the Levant
PART USED: Gum-resin
ACTION: Stimulant, resolvent
DISSERTATION: For ages it has been used internally in hysteria, rheumatism and chronic affections of the mucous air passages. Externally it is used in making plasters and ointments.
METHOD: Emulsion
DOSAGE: 10-30 gr.

CHRONIC BRONCHITIS AND CATARRH

PLANT: Iceland Moss *Cetraria islandica*
WHERE FOUND: Sweden, Central Europe
PART USED: Moss

ACTION: Demulcent, nutritive, tonic

DISSERTATION: Normal dosage to improve both appetite and digestion. It does not cause constipation, but heavy usage may induce looseness of the bowels.

METHOD: Decoction of 1 oz. well washed moss to 1 pt. water

DOSAGE: 1 to 4 oz.

CHRONIC CONSTIPATION — INTESTINAL INDIGESTION

PLANT: Black Root   *Leptandra virginica*

WHERE FOUND: North America

PART USED: Rhizome

ACTION: Antiseptic, cathartic, diaphoretic, tonic

DISSERTATION: Used mainly for its cathartic effect, for it acts with certainty and without griping. Invaluable in fevers, purifying the blood and removing morbid obstructions in a mild natural manner.

METHOD: Powder

DOSAGE: ¼ to 1 dr.

CHRONIC DISCHARGES OF BLOOD FROM THE UTERUS

PLANT: Saffron (Fall blooming)   *Crocus sativus*

WHERE FOUND: Asia Minor

PART USED: Flower pistils

ACTION: Carminative, diaphoretic, emmenagogue

DISSERTATION: It arrests chronic discharges of blood from the uterus. Also used in amenorrhoea, dysmenorrhoea and hysteria.

Saffron is mentioned once in the Bible in the Song of Solomon IV, 14, where Solomon places it in his garden of

sweets thus: "Spikenard and saffron; calamus and cinnamon, with all trees of frankincense."
METHOD: Infusion of 1 dr. in 1 pt. boiling water
DOSAGE: Given in wineglassful to teacupful doses

CHRONIC IRRITATION OF THE MUCOUS MEMBRANE

PLANT: Mountain Laurel   *Kalmia latifolia*
WHERE FOUND: United States
PART USED: Leaves
ACTION: Alterative, astringent, cardiac sedative
DISSERTATION: It is regarded as a most efficient remedy in overcoming obstinate chronic irritation of the mucous membrane.
METHOD: Decoction of 1 oz. of herb in 1 qt. water, boiled down to 1 pt.
DOSAGE: Tablespoonful doses

CHRONIC RHEUMATISM

PLANT: Guaiacum   *Guaiacum officinale*
WHERE FOUND: West Indies and South America
PART USED: Wood and resin
ACTION: Alterative, diaphoretic
DISSERTATION: It is considered a valuable remedy for chronic rheumatism, gout and impurities in the blood. It is generally used in conjunction with sarsaparilla and is used in most blood-purifying compounds.
METHOD: Infusion of 1 oz. to 1 pt. boiling water
DOSAGE: Tablespoonful 3 or 4 times a day

CHRONIC SCROFULOUS AND DYSPEPTIC COMPLAINTS

PLANT: May Apple or American Mandrake

Podophyllum peltatum

WHERE FOUND: North America

PART USED: Rhizome and the resin extracted from it

ACTION: Antibilious, cathartic, hydragogue, purgative

DISSERTATION: Mandrake is a powerful medicine, exercising an influence on every part of the system, stimulating the glands to a healthy action. Its most beneficial action is obtained by the use of small doses frequently given, as large ones cause violent evacuations and debility. In all chronic scrofulous and dyspeptic complaints it is highly valuable; also in dropsy, biliousness and liver disorders.

METHOD: Powdered root

DOSAGE: 2 to 10 gr.

Preparations of the root are to be preferred to those of the resin. This is one of the many illustrations of the fact that isolated principles do not act so well as in their natural position where they are associated with other remedial factors.

COMMON COLD AND COLD SORES

PLANT: Dulse, True and Common

Halymenia edulis and palmata

WHERE FOUND: Coast of Britain and New Brunswick

PART USED: Whole plant

ACTION: Corrective, deobstruent, depurative, nutritive, tonic, stimulant

DISSERTATION: Does not induce thirst. One of the best

33

balanced vegetable foods available. It is claimed that it contains more than 300 times more iodine than wheat and 50 times more iron.

For the treatment of colds and cold sores, its success is remarkable. Also a preventive of goitre.

METHOD: Eat the dried dulse as you would a stick of celery or a few leaves of lettuce

DOSAGE: About half an ounce daily

This is the best and the most edible of seaweeds. Most people regard it as a delicacy. In fact, Scots and Maritimers consider it a necessity.

COMPLEXION IMPROVER

PLANT: Goa, Araroba or Chrysarobin   *Andira araroba*
WHERE FOUND: Brazil
PART USED: Yellowish powder found in tree trunks
ACTION: Alterative, detergent, taenifuge
DISSERTATION: European healers have used it, because it contains chrysophanic acid, in skin diseases such as eczema, psoriasis and acne.
METHOD: The Goa powder is mixed with vinegar, lemon juice or glycerine to form a paste. It is also used as an ointment.
DOSAGE: Applied to skin as a paste

CONGESTIVE CHILLS AND INDIGESTION

PLANT: Pepper or Black Pepper   *Piper nigrum*
WHERE FOUND: Malabar and Travancore; also introduced to all other tropical areas
PART USED: Unripe berries
ACTION: Carminative, stimulant
DISSERTATION: Pepper is considered a valuable gastro-intestinal stimulant, of great service in flatulence, congestive chills and indigestion.
METHOD: Powdered peppercorns
DOSAGE: 3-15 gr.

CONSTIPATION

PLANT: Cassia Pods   *Cassia fistula*
WHERE FOUND: East and West Indies, Egypt
PART USED: Pulp
ACTION: Pleasant fruit laxative
DISSERTATION: Joseph Miller states: "The pulp of Cassia is a gentle, soluble medicine, pleasant to take and purges very gently, without gripings..."
      It is usually combined with Senna or some other laxative.
DOSAGE: 60 to 120 gr.

CONSTIPATION DUE TO INACTIVITY OF THE LIVER

PLANT: Wahoo   *Euonymus atropurpureus*
WHERE FOUND: North America
PART USED: Bark and bark of root
ACTION: Alterative, cholagogue, laxative, tonic
DISSERTATION: Valuable in liver disorders, especially those following or accompanied by fever. It may be given with every

confidence for constipation due to inactivity of liver.
METHOD: Ext. Euonym. B.P.C. 1949
DOSAGE: 1 to 2 gr.

CONVALESCENT FOOD

PLANT: Pot Barley   *Hordeum distichon*
WHERE FOUND: Worldwide, but native to Asia
PART USED: Seeds
ACTION: Demulcent, nutritive
DISSERTATION: For children suffering from diarrhoea, catarrhal inflammation of bowels. One of the world's oldest and most widely used foods, especially in the Northern hemisphere.
METHOD: Decoction of 2 oz. of washed barleycorns in one pint of water
DOSAGE: Take as desired

COUGH REMEDY

PLANT: Coltsfoot   *Tussilago farfara*
WHERE FOUND: Europe and Britain; grows in wet places and near brooks and rivers
PART USED: Leaves and flowers
ACTION: Demulcent, expectorant, pectoral
DISSERTATION: Esteemed as the most popular of cough remedies. Generally used with other herbs such as Horehound, Marshmallow, Ground Ivy and others.
METHOD: Decoction of 1 oz. leaves to 1 qt. water, boiled down to 1 pt.

DOSAGE: Teacupfuls sweetened with honey. The dried leaves, cut and rolled, are smoked like cigarettes in pulmonary conditions.

COUGH REMEDY

PLANT: Stramonium   *Datura stramonium*
WHERE FOUND: Europe
PART USED: Leaves and seeds
ACTION: Anodyne, antispasmodic, narcotic
DISSERTATION: It acts similar to Belladonna, but does not constipate. The inhalation from the smoke of burning leaves is recommended for relieving attacks of asthma.
METHOD: Extract Stramon. Liq. B.P.
DOSAGE: 1 to 3 min.

Old botanists claim it is a better cough remedy than opium, and it does not arrest secretions.

COUGHS, PAROXYSMAL, CONVULSIVE AND WHOOPING

PLANT: Chestnut   *Castanea sativa*
WHERE FOUND: Europe, Great Britain and America
PART USED: Leaves
ACTION: Astringent, tonic
DISSERTATION: In many lands chestnut leaves are quite popular in treatment for ague and fever. However it is best

known for its remedial benefits in paroxysmal or convulsive and whooping coughs, as well as other excitable and irritable ailments of the respiratory organs.

METHOD: Infusion of 1 oz. leaves in 1 pt. boiling water

DOSAGE: Tablespoonful to wineglassful doses, taken 3 to 4 times daily

COUNTERPOISON OF SERPENTS

PLANT: Rue or Ave-grace   *Ruta graveolens*

WHERE FOUND: Southern Europe and Great Britain

PART USED: Herb

ACTION: Antispasmodic, emmenagogue, stimulant

DISSERTATION: Dioscorides writes that "a twelve pennyweight of the seed drunk in wine is a counterpoison of serpents, the stinging of Scorpions, Bees, Hornets and Wasps; and it is reported that if a man be anointed with the juice of the Rue these will not hurt him; and that the serpent is driven away at the smell thereof when it is burned; insomuch that when the weasel is to fight with the serpent she armeth herself by eating Rue, against the might of the Serpent."

Rue was believed to possess the merits of dispelling infection and to this day the old custom of strewing the courts with herbs (of which Rue is an ingredient) is maintained. It was also used in the exorcisms ordained by the Roman Catholic Church, hence the synonym Ave-grace.

CRICK IN THE NECK

PLANT: Purslane   *Portulaca oleracea*
WHERE FOUND: Europe
PART USED: Seed and herb
ACTION: Diuretic
DISSERTATION: Culpeper says: "The seed is more effectual than the herb, and is good to cool the heat and sharpness of urine. The seed bruised and boiled in wine, and given to children, expels the worms. The juice of the herb is effectual to all the purposes aforenamed; also to stay vomitings, and taken with sugar and honey, helps an old and dry cough, shortness of breath, and the phthisic, and stays immoderate thirst. The juice is good for inflammations and ulcers in the secret parts, as well as in the bowels, and hemorrhoids, when they have excoriations in them; the herb bruised and applied to the forehead and temples, allays excessive heat therein, that hinders rest and sleep; and applied to the eyes it takes away inflammation in them, those other parts where pushes wheals, pimples, St. Anthony's fire, and the like, break forth; if a little vinegar be put to it, and laid to the neck, with as much of gall and linseed together, it takes away the pains therein, and the crick in the neck."

CURE-ALL

PLANT: Lobelia   *Lobelia inflata*
WHERE FOUND: Eastern United States, but cultivated widely
PART USED: Herb and seed
ACTION: Anti-asthmatic, emetic, expectorant, diaphoretic, stimulant
DISSERTATION: Highly controversial plant. Some of the best authorities speak of it as one of the most beneficial plants to be

found anywhere; others claim it to be a poison. Consensus of opinion suggests it is a great gift to mankind if used in moderation and with care and common sense.

METHOD: Infusion of 1 oz. powdered herb in 1 pt. boiling water

DOSAGE: ½ to 1 wineglassful

One top authority calls it "one of the most valuable remedies ever discovered." Here I will mention some of its uses: as an emetic; for bronchial troubles, pulmonary complaints, removing mucus, croup, and whooping cough; especially valuable in asthma and bronchial spasms; highly rated in infantile cough and bronchitis; in liver and stomach troubles an emetic of Lobelia will remove all immediate obstruction; and when mixed with powdered Slippery Elm it forms a stimulating poultice for inflammations, ulcers and swellings.

CURE-ALL

PLANT: Horsetail   *Equisetum arvense*

WHERE FOUND: Grows most everywhere

PART USED: Herb

ACTION: Astringent, diuretic

DISSERTATION: Used in dropsy, gravel and kidney complaints. The ashes of the plant are said to be used for acidity of the stomach and dyspepsia.

Culpeper states that this plant belongs to Saturn and recommends it to "staunch bleeding either inward or outward."

METHOD: Liquid extract

DOSAGE: ¼ to 1 dr.

CUTANEOUS TUMOURS

PLANT: Sorrel   *Rumex acetosa*
WHERE FOUND: Europe
PART USED: Leaves
ACTION: Diuretic, refrigerant
DISSERTATION: The following preparation has been used in cutaneous tumours.
METHOD: Burnt Alum 1 dr; Citric Acid 2 dr; inspissated juice of Sorrel 1 oz; water to 10 oz.
DOSAGE: Applied as a paint

CYSTITIS

PLANT: Marshmallow   *Althaea officinalis*
WHERE FOUND: Europe and Great Britain
PART USED: Leaves and root
ACTION: Demulcent, emollient

DISSERTATION: In painful complaints of urinary organs and cystitis it exerts a relaxing effect upon the passages as well as acting as a curative. The powdered or crushed fresh roots make a good poultice, which may be relied upon to remove the most obstinate inflammation and prevent mortification. Its powers in this direction are so great that it has been termed Mortification Root. The addition of Slippery Elm is an advantage and it should be applied to the part as hot as can be borne, renewing poultice when dry.

METHOD: An infusion of 1 oz. leaves to 1 pt. boiling water

DOSAGE: Wineglassful doses taken frequently

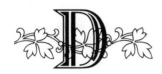

DIABETES

PLANT: Jambul   *Eugenia jambolana*
WHERE FOUND: East India, Australia
PART USED: Seeds
ACTION: Astringent, diuretic
DISSERTATION: These seeds have been found very useful in diabetes, as it reduces the amount of sugar present in urine in a comparatively short space of time. It must not be considered a specific in all cases of diabetes, but it does hold promise and can be of great value and should be given a trial.
METHOD AND DOSAGE: Van Noorden recommends large doses in cases of diabetes mellitus, and says ½ oz. of the fluid extract in 8 oz. of hot water should be taken one hour before breakfast and last thing at night.

DIABETES

PLANT: Periwinkle   *Vinca major*
WHERE FOUND: Southern Europe, and a widely distributed garden plant
PART USED: Herb
ACTION: Astringent, tonic

DISSERTATION: Joseph Miller describes it as "a good vulnerary plant, and of frequent use in wound-drinks..."

Vinca rosea, a fairly common, pinkish-white-flowered plant growing in South Africa, has been used by the natives for many years as a cure for diabetes. It is said to be more efficacious than Insulin. A registration officer in Durban was declared cured after two months' treatment, and considerable notice appeared in the South African and London Press as to its virtues.

DIABETES AND ASTHMA

PLANT: Jaborandi   *Pilocarpus microphyllus*
WHERE FOUND: Brazil
PART USED: Leaves
ACTION: Diaphoretic, expectorant, stimulant
DISSERTATION: Considered specially useful in diabetes and asthma.
METHOD: Infusion of 1 oz. leaves to 1 pt. boiling water
DOSAGE: Frequent mouthfuls

DIARRHOEA AND DYSENTERY

PLANT: Blackberry, American   *Rubus villosus*
WHERE FOUND: North America; also in Europe
PART USED: Root and leaves
ACTION: Astringent, tonic

DISSERTATION: A valuable remedy for diarrhoea and dysentery.
METHOD: Infusion of 1 oz. root or leaves to 1 pt. water
DOSAGE: Taken in wineglassful doses

DIM EYESIGHT AND FILMS THAT GROW OVER THE EYES
(Cataract)

PLANT: Willow, White   *Salix alba*
WHERE FOUND: Europe, Central Asia, North Africa
PART USED: Bark, leaves
ACTION: Antiperiodic, astringent, tonic
DISSERTATION: Parkinson writes: "The water that is gathered from the willow while it flowereth, the bark being slit and a vessel apt to receive it, being fitted to it, is very good for redness and dim eyesight and films that begin to grow over them..."

Also Parkinson: "The decoction of the leaves and bark in wine is good to bathe . . . the places pained with the gout . . . and to cleanse the head or other parts of scurfe... The juice of the leaves and green bark mingled with some Rosewater and heated in the rind of a pomegranet is singular good to help deafness to be dropped into the ears."

DIMMING VISION AND EYE INFLAMMATION

PLANT: Cornflower   *Centaurea cyanus*
WHERE FOUND: Found growing wild in cornfields; also common garden plant
PART USED: Flowers
ACTION: Stimulant and tonic
DISSERTATION: Eau de Casselunette, which means "break-spectacle water," was used in Paris in years gone by. Said to be an excellent remedy for the inflammation of the eyes and dimness of eyesight.
METHOD: Infusion of 1 oz. to 1 pt. water
DOSAGE: Wineglassful as required

DIPHTHERIA AND CROUP

PLANT: Papaya   *Carica papaya*
WHERE FOUND: Native to tropical America, but now grown in all tropical lands
PART USED: Papain, prepared from the juice of the unripe fruit and leaves
ACTION: Digestive
DISSERTATION: The digestive enzyme papain is administered widely in various digestive disorders where albuminoid substances pass away undigested. It is generally used in combination with an alkali, such as bicarbonate of soda, and acts best in an alkaline medium. A solution of the enzyme (ferment) is claimed to dissolve the false membranes in diphtheria and croup, when applied frequently.
METHOD: Papain
DOSAGE: 2 to 10 gr.

DROPSY

PLANT: Toadflax, Yellow   *Linaria vulgaris*
WHERE FOUND: Europe
PART USED: Herb
ACTION: Astringent, detergent, hepatic
DISSERTATION: A good application for piles is an ointment made from the fresh plant. As an alterative in jaundice, liver, skin diseases and scrofula. The old writers considered it a powerful diuretic, cathartic and deobstruent. It was therefore recommended by Tragus to carry off the water of dropsies and to remove obstructions of the liver.
METHOD: Infusion of 1 oz. herb to 1 pt. boiling water
DOSAGE: Take wineglassful doses as desired

DRUNKENNESS

PLANT: Wood Betony   *Stachys betonica*
WHERE FOUND: Europe
PART USED: Herb
ACTION: Alterative, aromatic, astringent
DISSERTATION: Parkinson states: ". . . it is said also to hinder drunkenness being taken beforehand and quickly to expel it afterwards . . ."
    The root is not used in medicine. It has an obnoxious flavor and induces vomiting.

DRY COUGHS

PLANT: Licorice or Liquorice   *Glycyrrhiza glabra*
WHERE FOUND: Mediterranean Europe
PART USED: Root
ACTION: Demulcent, emollient, pectoral
DISSERTATION: Here is a recipe used with much success by one Dr. Malone of London:

Take a large teaspoonful of Linseed, 1 oz. of Liquorice Root, and ¼ lb. of best raisins. Put them into 2 quarts of soft water and simmer down to 1 quart. Then add to it ¼ lb. brown sugar candy and tablespoonful of white wine vinegar or lemon juice. Drink ½ pint when going to bed and take a little whenever the cough is troublesome.

N.B. It is best to add the vinegar to that quantity which is required for immediate use.

DRYNESS AND ROUGHNESS OF TONGUE AND THROAT

PLANT: Flea-Wort　　　　　　　　　　*Erigeron viscosum*
WHERE FOUND: Britain
PART USED: Herb, seeds
ACTION: Aromatic, astringent, bitter
DISSERTATION: Culpeper states: "The seed dried, and taken, stays the flux or lax of the belly, and the corrosions that come by reason of hot choleric, or sharp and malignant humours, or by too much purging of any violent medicine, as scammony, or the like. The mucilage of the seed made with rose water, and a little sugar-candy put thereto, is very good in all hot agues and burning fevers, and other inflammations, to cool thirst, and lenify the dryness and roughness of the tongue and throat. It helps all hoarseness of the voice, and diseases of the breast and lungs, caused by heat, or sharp salt humours, and the pleurisy also."

DYSENTERY

PLANT: Bael　　　　　　　　　　*Aegle marmelos*
WHERE FOUND: India
PART USED: Fruit, unripe and dried
ACTION: Astringent, laxative
DISSERTATION: This is an Indian remedy and is considered practically a specific for diarrhoea and dysentery in that country. It is claimed that it never constipates.
METHOD: Liquid extract. Also used in the form of a decoction or jelly.
DOSAGE: 60-120 min.

DYSMENORRHOEA (Painful)

PLANT: Pulsatilla   *Anemone pulsatilla*
WHERE FOUND: Europe and Asia
PART USED: Herb
ACTION: Alterative, antispasmodic, nervine
DISSERTATION: Highly valued as a remedy for nerve exhaustion in women, especially when due to menstrual difficulties. Has a stimulating effect on all mucus surfaces. Valuable in catarrh, amenorrhoea and other conditions.
METHOD: Fluid extract
DOSAGE: 2 to 5 drops every few hours during the day prior to the expected period

DYSPEPSIA

PLANT: Centaury   *Erythraea centaurium*
WHERE FOUND: Europe and British heaths
PART USED: Herb, leaves
ACTION: Aromatic, bitter, stomachic, tonic
DISSERTATION: Most used in dyspepsia. Also used in conjunction with Barberry bark for jaundice.
  Culpeper writes: "The herb is so safe you cannot fail in using of it. Take it inwardly only for inward diseases, and apply it outwardly for outward complaints; it is very wholesome, but not pleasant to the taste."
METHOD: Infusion of 1 oz. to 1 pt. boiling water
DOSAGE: Wineglassful as desired

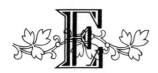

ECZEMA

PLANT: Celandine   *Chelidonium majus*
WHERE FOUND: Europe and English gardens
PART USED: Herb
ACTION: Alterative, diuretic, purgative
DISSERTATION: Long used for eczema, scrofulous diseases, jaundice. The fresh juice is excellent when applied to corns and warts.
METHOD: Infusion of 1 oz. herb to 1 pt. boiling water
DOSAGE: Wineglassful doses as needed

ELEPHANTIASIS

PLANT: Calotropis   *Calotropis procera*
WHERE FOUND: India
PART USED: Bark
ACTION: Sudorific, tonic
DISSERTATION: In India it is used as a local remedy for elephantiasis, leprosy and chronic eczema. Internally for diarrhoea and dysentery.
METHOD: Powdered bark
DOSAGE: 3 to 10 gr. as an expectorant

51

ELIXIR

PLANT: Slippery Elm   *Ulmus fulva*
WHERE FOUND: North and Central America
PART USED: Inner bark
ACTION: Demulcent, diuretic, emollient, pectoral
DISSERTATION: The food or gruel should be made as follows:
Take a teaspoonful of the powder, mix well with the same
quantity of powdered sugar and add 1 pt. of boiling water
slowly, mixing as it is poured on. This may be flavoured with
cinnamon or nutmeg to suit the taste, and makes a very
wholesome and sustaining food for infants.

The coarse powder forms the finest poultice to be
obtained for all inflamed surfaces, ulcers, wounds, burns, boils,
skin diseases, purulent ophthalmia, chilblains, etc. It soothes the
part, disperses the inflammation, draws out impurities, and
heals speedily.

We cannot speak too highly of this remedy, and are
confident there is nothing to equal it in the world for its
above-mentioned uses.
METHOD AND DOSAGE: Inflammation in the bowels of
infants and adults has been cured, when all other remedies have
failed, by an injection into the bowels of an infusion of 1 oz. of
powdered bark to 1 pt. of boiling water, used while warm.

Said to be one of the most valuable materials in the
botanic practice. The finely powdered inner bark makes an
excellent food and can be used in all cases of weakness,
inflammation of the stomach, and bronchitis. It has a soothing
healing action on all parts of contact and it is claimed to be as
nutritive as oatmeal.

ENERGESIS

PLANT: Yerba Mate or Paraguay Tea   *Ilex paraguensis*
WHERE FOUND: Paraguay, Brazil and other South American countries
PART USED: Leaves, and also the finely ground stems
ACTION: Diuretic, stimulant
DISSERTATION: It is claimed that the natives can do a real hard day's work with nothing but frequent cups of strong Mate. General action similar to coffee or tea but much more stimulating, so its users claim. Does have anti-scorbutic qualities. Recommended for rheumatism and gout.
METHOD: Infusion as tea — a teaspoonful to a cup of boiling water
DOSAGE: Take as desired

ENFEEBLED STOMACH AND INTESTINES

PLANT: Canella   *Canella alba*
WHERE FOUND: West Indies
PART USED: Bark
ACTION: Antiscorbutic, aromatic, stimulant, tonic
DISSERTATION: Useful in enfeebled conditions of the stomach and intestines. Used as a condiment by the natives in the West Indies.
METHOD: Pulverized bark
DOSAGE: 3 to 10 gr.

ENLARGED PROSTATE, SPERMATORRHOEA, ABORTION

PLANT: Ergot   *Claviceps purpurea*
WHERE FOUND: Wherever rye is grown
PART USED: Fungus

ACTION: Emmenagogue, haemostatic, uterine stimulant

DISSERTATION: Considered of value in enlarged prostate and spermatorrhoea. Has been widely used for many years in menstrual disorders, leucorrhoea, dysmenorrhoea, amenorrhoea and for its notable stimulating action. Also esteemed for haemorrhage, flooding and intestinal bleeding.

METHOD: Liquid extract of Ergot

DOSAGE: 10 to 20 min.

ENLARGEMENT OF SPLEEN

PLANT: Hedge-Hyssop   *Gratiola officinalis*

WHERE FOUND: Boggy places in the English countryside

PART USED: Herb, root

ACTION: Cathartic, diuretic, emetic

DISSERTATION: Recommended in enlargement of the spleen, chronic affections of the liver and jaundice. It has also proven itself valuable in dropsical affections. Large doses induce vomiting and purging.

METHOD: Infusion of ½ oz. powdered root to 1 pt. boiling water

DOSAGE: Tablespoonful doses as indicated

EYE DISEASES

PLANT: Quince   *Cydonia oblongata*

WHERE FOUND: Persia, but planted in Europe and America

PART USED: Seeds

ACTION: Demulcent, mucilaginous

DISSERTATION: Externally it is used in eye diseases as a soothing lotion.

Culpeper recommends the fruit juice as a preservative against the force of deadly poisons . . . "For it hath been found most true that the very smell of a quince hath taken away all the strength of the poison of white hellebore."

EYE DISORDERS

PLANT: Eyebright   *Euphrasia officinalis*
WHERE FOUND: Europe and Britain
PART USED: Herb
ACTION: Astringent and slightly tonic
DISSERTATION: Its principal use is in treatment of the eyes: diseases of sight, weakness of vision and ophthalmia. An excellent lotion for general disorders of the eye is made in combination with Golden Seal.

Culpeper states: "If the herb was but as much used as it is neglected, it would spoil the spectacle makers' trade; and a man would think, that reason should teach people to prefer the preservation of their natural before artificial spectacles; which that they may be instructed how to do, take the virtues of Eyebright as follows —

The juice or distilled water of the Eyebright taken inwardly in white wine or broth or dropped into the eyes for divers days together, helps all infirmities of the eyes that cause dimness of sight."
METHOD: Liquid extract
DOSAGE: 1 dr.

EYE TROUBLES

PLANT: Clary   *Salvia sclarea*
WHERE FOUND: Found throughout Europe and the British Isles
PART USED: Herb, seed
ACTION: Antispasmodic and balsamic
DISSERTATION: It is most useful and efficacious in any complaint of the eyes. Has also given relief in kidney diseases. Valued also as a stomachic in digestive troubles.

Parkinson writes: "The fresh leaves fried in butter, being first dipped in a batter of flour, eggs and a little milk served as a dish to the table is not unpleasant to any ..." Also: "Some brewers of ale and beer do put it into their drink to make it more heady, fit to please drunkards who thereby become either dead drunk or foolish drunk or mad drunk."
METHOD: Decoction of 1 oz. herb to 1 pt. boiling water
DOSAGE: Wineglassful twice daily

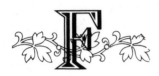

FALLING SICKNESS

PLANT: Peony   *Paeonia officinalis*
WHERE FOUND: China and Tibet, but today a common and
beautiful garden flower
PART USED: Root
ACTION: Antispasmodic, tonic
DISSERTATION: Culpeper describes it as a herb of the Sun
and under the lion. He recommends it for the falling sickness
(epilepsy) and states "but the surest way is (besides hanging it
about the neck, by which children have been cured) to take the
root of the male peony washed clean and stamped small and
infuse it in sack for twenty-four hours at least; afterwards strain
it, and take, morning and evening, a good draught for sundry
days together before and after a full moon . . ."

FALLING SICKNESS

PLANT: Parsley   *Carum petroselinum*
WHERE FOUND: Eastern Mediterranean countries, but found
in most gardens
PART USED: Root, seed, leaves
ACTION: Aperient, diuretic, emmenagogue

DISSERTATION: Parkinson writes: "Tragus setteth downe an excellent medicine to help the jaundices and falling sickness, the Dropsie and stone in Reynes or Kidneyes in this manner; take saith he of the seeds of Parsley, Fennell, Anise and Caraways, of each an ounce, of the roots of Parsley, Burnet, Saxifrage and Caraways, of each one ounce and a halfe; let the seeds be bruised and the rootes washed and cut small; let them all lye in steepe in a pottle of white wine, and in the morning boyled in a close earthen vessell until a third part or more be wasted, which being strained and cleared take four ounces thereof at a time, morning and evening first and last, abstaining from drink for three houres after ..."

FEBRILE DISEASES

PLANT: Tamarinds   *Tamarindus indica*
WHERE FOUND: Native to central Africa; cultivated in West Indies, India and East Indies
PART USED: Fruit, pulp
ACTION: Laxative, nutritive, refrigerant
DISSERTATION: Considered an agreeable refrigerating drink in febrile diseases when used in small quantities and diluted with water. Also form a part of confection of Senna.
METHOD: 1 oz. pulp boiled in 1 pt. milk and then strained
DOSAGE: 2 to 4 drams

Joseph Miller writes: "They are accounted specific for all disorders of the Spleen, as being believed to lessen it much; nay they used to drink out of cups made of this wood to cure those illnesses."

FEVERS

PLANT: Balm   *Melissa officinalis*
WHERE FOUND: Widely planted in gardens, but native to Eurasia
PART USED: Herb
ACTION: Carminative, diaphoretic, febrifuge
DISSERTATION: Induces mild perspiration, and also makes a pleasant and cooling tea for feverish patients. Considered a most useful herb either alone or in combination with others.
METHOD: 1 oz. herb in 1 pt. boiling water, allow to cool and then strain
DOSAGE: Drink freely

FEVERS (Intermittent)

PLANT: Berberis   *Berberis aristata*
WHERE FOUND: Native to India
PART USED: Stem
ACTION: Febrifuge, tonic
DISSERTATION: Used in India as a bitter tonic in intermittent fevers.
METHOD: Powder
DOSAGE: 10 to 60 gr.

FEVERS (Including Malaria)

PLANT: Cinchona   *Cinchona officinalis*
WHERE FOUND: The Andes in South America
PART USED: Bark
ACTION: Antiperiodic, astringent, febrifuge, tonic

DISSERTATION: A much esteemed herb in all typhoid and febrile conditions, and also for remittent and intermittent fevers. Highly rated as a general tonic and in debility, dyspepsia and neuralgia.
METHOD: Powdered bark
DOSAGE: 5 to 15 gr.

FILLING FOR CARIOUS TEETH

PLANT: Mastic   *Pistacia lentiscus*
WHERE FOUND: Grecian Archipelago, Cyprus
PART USED: Resin
ACTION: Filling agent
DISSERTATION: The resin by itself or in a spirituous solution is used in dentistry as a filling for carious teeth.

FISTULA

PLANT: Agrimony   *Agrimonia eupatoria*
WHERE FOUND: Europe
PART USED: Herb
ACTION: Deobstruent, diuretic, mild astringent, tonic
DISSERTATION: John Parkinson in the Theater of Plants (1640) recommends that a decoction of the plant "made with wine and drunk, is good against the sting and biting of Serpents." Outwardly applied, a decoction in wine "... doth draw forth the thorns and splinters of wood, nails, or any other such thing that is gotten into the flesh..."

FOOD FROM HEAVEN

PLANT: Manna   *Fraxinus ornus*
WHERE FOUND: Southern Europe
PART USED: Concrete exudation
ACTION: Laxative, nutritive
DISSERTATION: Considered useful as a laxative for infants, children and pregnant women.
METHOD: Combined with a laxative or carminative
DOSAGE: Teaspoonful up to 2 oz.

FRECKLES, SPOTS AND PIMPLES ON THE FACE

PLANT: Silverweed   *Potentilla anserina*
WHERE FOUND: Europe and Great Britain
PART USED: Herb
ACTION: Astringent, tonic
DISSERTATION: Gerard writes: "The distilled water takes away freckles, spots, pimples in the face, and sun-burning, but the herb, laid to infuse or steep in white wine is far better: but the best of all is to steep it in strong white wine vinegar, the face being often bathed or washed therewith."

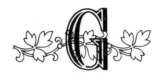

GALL STONES

PLANT: Fringetree   *Chionanthus virginica*
WHERE FOUND: Southern United States
PART USED: Bark of root
ACTION: Alterative, diuretic, tonic
DISSERTATION: It acts quickly and efficaciously in liver derangements as well as in jaundice and gall stones. In female disorders it is beneficial in conjunction with Pulsatilla and other remedies.
METHOD: Infusion of 1 oz. to 1 pt. boiling water. May be used externally as a lotion or injection.
DOSAGE: Tablespoonful to wineglassful doses, as suited

GANGRENE AND MORTIFICATION PREVENTIVE

PLANT: Wood Sage   *Teucrium scorodonia*
WHERE FOUND: Europe and Asia
PART USED: Herb
ACTION: Astringent, diaphoretic, emmenagogue, tonic
DISSERTATION: Joseph Miller recommends this herb for gout and rheumatism and also as a vulnerary plant, stating that it prevents mortification and gangrene.

METHOD: Infusion of 1 oz. herb in 1 pt. boiling water
DOSAGE: Wineglassful doses

GASTRIC IRRITATION AND CONGESTION

PLANT: Peach   *Prunus persica*
WHERE FOUND: Native to Persia and China, now widely grown
PART USED: Bark, leaves and oil pressed from the seeds
ACTION: Diuretic, expectorant, sedative
DISSERTATION: It has been found almost a specific for irritation and congestion of gastric surfaces. Used also in coughs, whooping cough and chronic bronchitis.
METHOD: Infusion of ½ oz. of bark or 1 oz. of leaves to 1 pt. of boiling water
DOSAGE: Teaspoonful to a wineglassful as desired

GLANDULAR ENLARGEMENT

PLANT: Ivy   *Hedera helix*
WHERE FOUND: Native to Europe and Britain, but grown in most gardens
PART USED: Leaves, berries
ACTION: Cathartic, diaphoretic, stimulant
DISSERTATION: Externally the leaves have been employed as poultices or fomentations in glandular enlargements, indolent ulcers and abscesses. It is claimed that a vinegar of these berries was used extensively during the London plague.

GNAWING OF THE HEART

PLANT: Spearmint *Mentha viridis*
WHERE FOUND: Worldwide
PART USED: Herb, oil
ACTION: Antispasmodic, carminative, hepatic, stimulant
DISSERTATION: Excellent for adding to other herbs to improve both their action and flavor.

Culpeper writes: "It helps a cold liver, strengthens the belly, causes digestion, stays vomiting and the hiccough; it is good against the gnawing of the heart, provokes appetite, takes away obstructions of the liver, but too much must not be taken, because it makes the blood thin, and turns it into choler, therefore choleric persons must abstain from it."
METHOD: Infusion of 1 oz. to 1 pt. boiling water. Sweeten with honey for infants.
DOSAGE: Wineglassful doses or less, as needed

Thomas Green states in his Universal Herbal: "The distilled water, or infusion, is much used in crudities and weaknesses of the stomach, heaving or retchings, hiccup, windiness and burning heat. It is likewise good in griping pains of the stomach and bowels, and in giddiness and swimmings of the head. Applied externally, it takes away hardness of the breasts, and cures the headache. A strong decoction is an excellent wash for eruptions on the skin, chaps, and sore heads."

GONORRHEA, GLEET, LEUCORRHOEA

PLANT: Copaiba   *Copaifera langsdorffii*
WHERE FOUND: Brazil and north of South America
PART USED: Oleoresin
ACTION: Cathartic, diuretic, stimulant
DISSERTATION: First introduced into Europe in the 17th century. Useful in excessive mucous discharges such as encountered in chronic catarrh of the bladder, gleet and leucorrhoea. Has very harsh taste; thus it is generally given in capsule form in combination with Santal Oil, Cubebs, or others.
METHOD: Oil Copaib. (The tree is tapped to obtain the oleoresin)
DOSAGE: 5 to 10 min.

GOUT AND RHEUMATISM

PLANT: Birthwort   *Aristolochia longa*
WHERE FOUND: Europe
PART USED: Root
ACTION: Aromatic, stimulant
DISSERTATION: Said by Joseph Miller, a famous herbalist, "Cleanses the stomach and lungs of tough phlegm ... outwardly it is useful in cleansing sordid ulcers."
METHOD: Powdered root
DOSAGE: ½ to 1 dr.

Dioscorides states of Birthwort that the powder being drunk in wine "brings away both birth and afterbirth and whatsoever a careless midwife hath left behind."

GRANULAR CONJUNCTIVITIS

PLANT: Poke Root   *Phytolacca decandra*
WHERE FOUND: North America
PART USED: Root, berries
ACTION: Alterative, cathartic, emetic
DISSERTATION: It has for many years been used in the treatment of granular conjunctivitis. Also considered a valuable remedy in scabies, ulcers, ringworm, chronic rheumatism, dysmenorrhoea and dyspepsia. The berries are considered milder in action than the root.
METHOD AND DOSAGE: Liquid extract, berries — ½ to 1 dr; Powdered root — 1 to 5 gr

GRAVEL AND DROPSY

PLANT: Bilberry   *Vaccinium myrtillus*
WHERE FOUND: Europe; likes boggy locations
PART USED: Ripe fruits
ACTION: Astringent, diuretic, refrigerant
DISSERTATION: Of proven benefit in dropsy and gravel.
METHOD: Decoction of 1 oz. in 1 pt. boiling water
DOSAGE: Taken in tablespoonful or wineglassful doses as required

GRAVES DISEASE (Erophthalmic Goitre)

PLANT: Speedwell   *Veronica officinalis*
WHERE FOUND: Europe
PART USED: Herb
ACTION: Alterative, diuretic, expectorant

DISSERTATION: Especially recommended in Graves disease and nephritis, opens all obstructions, promotes the menses. Known as a remedy against coughs, asthma and lung diseases.
METHOD: Infusion of 2 oz. in 1 pt. boiling water
DOSAGE: Small wineglassful doses as required

GREEN WOUNDS

PLANT: Knapweed   *Centaurea nigra*
WHERE FOUND: Native to Great Britain and Europe
PART USED: Herb
ACTION: Diaphoretic, diuretic, tonic
DISSERTATION: It is regarded as highly as Gentian as a tonic.
        Culpeper says: "It is an admirable remedy for a sore throat, swelling of the uvula and jaw, and all green wounds."

GUM STRENGTHENER

PLANT: Water Dock   *Rumex aquaticus*
WHERE FOUND: Europe
PART USED: Root
ACTION: Alterative, deobstruent, detergent
DISSERTATION: Valuable remedy for cleansing ulcers of the mouth. As a powder it has detergent effects on the teeth. The root finely powdered has been recommended as an excellent dentifrice to strengthen the gums.
METHOD: Infusion of 1 oz. root to 1 pt. boiling water
DOSAGE: Wineglassful doses

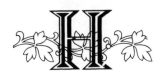

HAY FEVER AND ASTHMA

PLANT: Ephedra or Ma Huang　　　　　*Ephedra sinica*
WHERE FOUND: Northern China
PART USED: Stems
ACTION: Reduces susceptability to hay fever and asthma
DISSERTATION: It is claimed to have been used by the Chinese for thousands of years for asthmatic afflictions and bouts of hay fever. Ephedrine, the alkaloid, is the chief constituent.
METHOD: Liquid extract of Ephedrine
DOSAGE: ¼ to 1 dr.

HEAD WASH

PLANT: Foenugreek　　　　　*Trigonella foenum-graecum*
WHERE FOUND: North Africa and India
PART USED: Seeds
ACTION: Emollient
DISSERTATION: Used externally as a poultice in abscesses, boils and carbuncles. Taken internally for inflamed conditions of stomach and intestines.
METHOD: Decoction of 1 oz. of seeds in 1 pt. water

69

DOSAGE: Teacupful doses as desired

Gerard says: "It is good to wash the head with the decoction of the seed, for it taketh away the scurf, scales, nits, and all other such like imperfections."

HEART DISORDERS

PLANT: Hawthorn   *Crataegus oxycantha*
WHERE FOUND: Grows wild in woodlands in America and Great Britain
PART USED: Dried berries
ACTION: Cardiac, tonic
DISSERTATION: These berries are claimed to be a curative remedy for organic and functional heart disorders such as dyspnoea, rapid and feeble heart action, hypertrophy, valvular insufficiency and heart oppression.
METHOD: Liquid extract
DOSAGE: 10 to 15 drops taken 3 or 4 times a day

HEART STRAIN

PLANT: Hellebore, False   *Adonis vernalis*
WHERE FOUND: North Europe and Asia
PART USED: Herb
ACTION: Cardiac, diuretic, tonic
DISSERTATION: **Must be used with caution!** Valuable remedy

for heart strain and dropsy. Highly referred to in heart diseases and kidney affections.

METHOD: Infusion of ¼ oz. herb in 1 pt. boiling water

DOSAGE: Tablespoonful every three hours

HEMORRHOIDAL SWELLINGS

PLANT: Mayweed   *Anthemis cotula*

WHERE FOUND: Europe; found growing among corn

PART USED: Herb

ACTION: Antispasmodic, emetic, emmenagogue, tonic

DISSERTATION: Used for sick headache, convalescence from fever and amenorrhoea.

John Miller states: "This is a plant, but rarely used, though some authors commend it as good against Vapours and Hysteric Fits. Mr. Ray says it is sometimes made use of in scrofulous cases: and Tournefort, That about Paris they use it in Fomentations for pains and swellings of the Haemorrhoides."

METHOD: Infusion of 1 oz. herb to 1 pt. boiling water

DOSAGE: Wineglassful doses as required.

HEPATIC TORPOR AND CATARRH OF THE BLADDER

PLANT: Boldo   *Peumus boldus*

WHERE FOUND: Chile

PART USED: Leaves

ACTION: Antiseptic, diuretic, liver stimulant

DISSERTATION: Used chiefly against rheumatic pains, gall and bladder conditions; also in chronic hepatic torpor and dyspepsia.

METHOD: Liquid extract

DOSAGE: 1/6 to 1/2 dr.

HOARSENESS

PLANT: Hedge Mustard   *Sisymbrium officinale*
WHERE FOUND: Europe and Great Britain
PART USED: Herb
ACTION: Cephalic, cooling, sedative
DISSERTATION: A remedy for hoarseness and weak lungs. It is claimed to be an excellent aid in recovering the voice.
METHOD: Liquid extract
DOSAGE: ½ to 1 fl. dr.

HYDROPHOBIA AND HYSTERIA

PLANT: Skullcap   *Scutellaria laterifolia*
WHERE FOUND: North America
PART USED: Herb
ACTION: Antispasmodic, astringent, nervine, tonic
DISSERTATION: Claimed by herbalists to be the finest nervine ever discovered. It is suggested that it be prescribed wherever disorders of the nervous system exist. Its action is invaluable in convulsions, hydrophobia, hysteria, rickets and St. Vitus Dance.
METHOD: Infusion of 1 oz. herb to 1 pt. boiling water
DOSAGE: Half a teacupful frequently.

Many cases of hydrophobia are known to have been cured by this remedy alone, while it may be regarded as a specific in St. Vitus Dance. Also used to lessen desire to masturbate.

HYPNOTIC EFFECT, TO ACHIEVE

PLANT: Lachnanthes or Spiritweed   *Lachnanthes tinctoria*
WHERE FOUND: West Indies
PART USED: Root, herb
ACTION: Hypnotic, stimulating
DISSERTATION: Large doses produce strange, unusual and unpleasant symptoms. Has been used for coughs.
METHOD: Liquid extract
DOSAGE: 1 to 5 min.

HYSTERIA AND NERVOUS AFFECTIONS (Female)

PLANT: Chamomile   *Anthemis nobilis*
WHERE FOUND: Belgium, France and England; and of broad distribution
PART USED: Herb and flowers
ACTION: Antispasmodic, stomachic, tonic
DISSERTATION: Very old renowned herb used for at least many centuries. Has been proven efficacious and is best known for its use in hysteria and nervous complaints of women. Makes a superior poultice when combined with crushed poppy heads, for relieving various pains and aches. Also used externally for neuralgia, toothache and earache.
METHOD: Infusion of 1 oz. to 1 pt. boiling water
DOSAGE: From a tablespoonful to a wineglassful

HYSTERICAL COMPLAINTS

PLANT: Camphor   *Cinnamomum camphora*
WHERE FOUND: Central China and Japan

PART USED: Distillation of Camphor wood chips
ACTION: Anodyne, anthelmintic, antispasmodic, diaphoretic, sedative
DISSERTATION: Internally it is used in cold chills. It has been found of great value in all inflammatory affections, fever and hysterical complaints. It also acts beneficially in gout, rheumatic pains and neuralgia. It is highly valued in all irritation of sexual organs. Externally, it can be safely applied in all cases of inflammation, bruises and sprains.
METHOD: Oil of Camphor
DOSAGE: 2 to 5 gr.

Joseph Miller writes: "Some people hang it in a silk bag, about the neck, to cure agues."

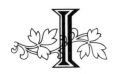

IMBALANCED DIET

PLANT: Kelp, Pacific   *Macrocystis pyrifera*
WHERE FOUND: Coast of California
PART USED: Whole plant
ACTION: Alterative, corrective, nutritive, tonic
DISSERTATION: Said to prevent common goitre. Also of value in its treatment; considered an excellent source of iodine. Dried kelp contains about ten times as much iodine as the same amount of iodized salt. An excellent substitute for salt. Contains a wide variety of elements and nutrients highly regarded by health-minded people.
METHOD: Used as a condiment as you would table salt
DOSAGE: Daily with meals

IMPOTENCE

PLANT: Nux Vomica   *Strychnos nux vomica*
WHERE FOUND: India, Burma, China, Australia
PART USED: Seeds
ACTION: Bitter, stimulant, tonic
DISSERTATION: Used as a general tonic, best in combination with other remedies. Useful in impotence, neuralgia, dyspepsia,

debility and chronic constipation, because it promotes peristalsis action.

    Caution: Must be used with great care for it is a poison. Nux Vomica was not used by the ancient herbalists as a medicine.

METHOD: Liquid Ext. Nuc. Vom. B.P.

DOSAGE: 1 to 3 min.

Parkinson and later Joseph Miller both mention its use in poisoning dogs, cats, crows and ravens.

IMPOTENCE AND IRRITATION OF URINARY ORGANS

PLANT: Burra Gokeroo   *Pedalium murex*

WHERE FOUND: India

PART USED: Seeds

ACTION: Antispasmodic, demulcent, diuretic

DISSERTATION: Has been used in incontinence of urine, gleet, nocturnal emissions, impotence and irritation of urinary organs.

METHOD: Infusion — 1 in 20

DOSAGE: Several doses each day

IMPURE BLOOD, BOILS, CARBUNCLES, GANGRENE

PLANT: Echinacea   *Echinacea angustifolia*

WHERE FOUND: Western prairies of America

PART USED: Rhizome

ACTION: Alterative, antiseptic
DISSERTATION: Useful in all diseases that are caused by impurities in the blood, such as boils, carbuncles and gangrene, both internally and externally. It improves the appetite and assists digestion. Beneficial in fermentative dyspepsia.
METHOD: Liquid extract
DOSAGE: ½ to 1 dr.

INCITE TO VENERY

PLANT: Wild Mint   *Mentha sativa*
WHERE FOUND: Europe, America
PART USED: Herb
ACTION: Astringent, emetic, stimulant
DISSERTATION: Useful herb in difficult menstruation and diarrhoea.

Parkinson writes: "Aristotle and others in the ancient times forbade Mints to be used of soldiers in the time of war, because they thought it did so much to incite to Venery, that it took away, or at least abated their animosity or courage to fight."
METHOD: Infusion of 1 oz. herb to 1 pt. boiling water
DOSAGE: Wineglassful doses

INFANTILE CONVULSIONS, TEETHING AND OTHER AILMENTS

PLANT: Chamomile, German   *Metricaria chamomilla*
WHERE FOUND: Most parts of Europe, the British Isles and elsewhere
PART USED: Flowers
ACTION: Carminative, sedative, tonic

DISSERTATION: Excellent remedy in children's ailments. Of benefit to the nerves (sedative) and tonic for the gastro-intestinal tract. Most useful during teething, for neuralgic pains, stomach upsets, earache and infantile convulsions.
METHOD: Infusion of ½ oz. to 1 pt. boiling water
DOSAGE: Give children freely in teaspoonful doses. Externally used as a poultice.

INFANTS' CORDIAL

PLANT: Peppermint   *Mentha piperita*
WHERE FOUND: All over Europe and North America
PART USED: Herb and oil (distilled)
ACTION: Carminative, stimulant, stomachic
DISSERTATION: An old remedy for allaying nausea, flatulence, sickness, vomiting and as an infants' cordial.
METHOD: Infusion of 1 oz. herb to 1 pt. boiling water
DOSAGE: Wineglassful doses

INFLAMMATORY DISEASES

PLANT: Abscess Root   *Polemonium reptans*
WHERE FOUND: Northern Europe
PART USED: Rhizome
ACTION: Alterative, astringent, diaphoretic, expectorant
DISSERTATION: Used in febrile, inflammatory diseases, pleurisy, coughs, colds, bronchial and lung disorders.
METHOD: Infusion of 1 oz. to 1 pt. boiling water
DOSAGE: Wineglassful doses, preferably warm

INGROWING TOENAILS

PLANT: Amadou   *Polyporus fomentarius*
WHERE FOUND: Europe and Great Britain
PART USED: A hoof-shaped, obliquely triangular, sessile fungus. The inner part is composed of short tubular fibres arranged in layers.
ACTION: Haemostatic, styptic
DISSERTATION: Amadou, known as Surgeon's Agaric, has been used for ages for arresting local haemorrhages. It is applied with pressure to the affected part.
METHOD: It is prepared for use by being cut into slices, chopped and beaten, soaked in a solution of nitre, and allowed to dry. Then insert it between the nail and flesh.

> When inserted between the nail and the flesh, it is one of the best known substances for treating ingrowing toenails.

INSOMNIA

PLANT: Gelsemium   *Gelsemium sempervirens*
WHERE FOUND: Southern United States
PART USED: Root
ACTION: Antispasmodic, arterial sedative, diaphoretic, febrifuge
DISSERTATION: When used in small doses it allays nervous excitement and irritation. Found useful in inflammation of the bowels, diarrhoea, dysentery and even with greater success in neuralgia, insomnia and toothache. Excellent wherever a

79

sedative is desired. Long a favorite remedy in female pelvic disorders. It is harmful in large doses and can depress the nervous system and give rise to convulsions and toxic symptoms.

METHOD: Tincture Gelsemium
DOSAGE: 5 to 15 drops

INTERMITTENT AND REMITTENT FEVERS

PLANT: Canadian Hemp *Apocynum cannabinum*
WHERE FOUND: North America
PART USED: Root and rhizome
ACTION: Diaphoretic, diuretic, emetic, expectorant
DISSERTATION: Valuable in cardiac dropsy. Recommended favorably in intermittent and remittent fevers. Useful in amenorrhoea and leucorrhoea.
METHOD: Decoction of 1 oz. to 1 pt. water
DOSAGE: Taken in tablespoonful doses frequently

INTESTINAL LUBRICANT

PLANT: Psyllium *Plantago psyllium*
WHERE FOUND: South Europe
PART USED: Seeds
ACTION: Mucilaginous, bulking agent
DISSERTATION: The seeds swell into a gelatinous mass when moistened, which stimulates and lubricates the intestinal tract.
METHOD: Place the psyllium in a glass and add warm water. Then stir until the mixture thickens, and then drink. Add a trace of fresh juice to make it palatable.
DOSAGE: Adult dose — 2 to 4 teaspoonfuls after meals

INTESTINAL WORMS

PLANT: Butternut   *Juglans cinerea*
WHERE FOUND: North America
PART USED: Inner bark
ACTION: Cathartic, tonic, vermifuge
DISSERTATION: A gentle purgative which does not bind after working. Also a remedy for worms in children
METHOD: Make a syrup of ½ oz. of extract to 8 oz. simple syrup, beating well together in a mortar
DOSAGE: 1 tablespoonful of syrup twice daily

INWARD AND OUTWARD WOUNDS

PLANT: Self-Heal   *Prunella vulgaris*
WHERE FOUND: Europe
PART USED: Herb
ACTION: Astringent
DISSERTATION: An old German saying is that "He needs neither physician nor surgeon that hath Self-Heal and to help himself."

> Culpeper writes: "Here is another herb of Venus, Self-Heal whereby when you are hurt you may heal yourself; it is a special herb for inward and outward wounds. Take it inwardly in syrups for inward wounds, outwardly in unguents and plaisters for outward... The juice thereof used with oil of roses to anoint the temples and forehead is very effectual to remove headache."

IRON DEFICIENCY (Chlorosis)

PLANT: Hellebore, Black or Christmas Rose   *Helleborus niger*
WHERE FOUND: Throughout most of Europe; cultivated in England
PART USED: Rhizome
ACTION: Cathartic, diuretic, emmenagogue
DISSERTATION: Has been used in chlorosis, amenorrhoea, and dropsy. Valuable in nervous disorders, hysteria and melancholia. Should be handled carefully and used only in minute doses.
METHOD: Liquid extract
DOSAGE: 2 to 10 min.

JAUNDICE, FEMALE OBSTRUCTIONS
AND SCROFULOUS TUMORS

PLANT: Butcher's Broom   *Ruscus aculeatus*
WHERE FOUND: In the thickets in Britain
PART USED: Root, herb
ACTION: Aperient, deobstruent, diaphoretic, diuretic, laxative, sudorific
DISSERTATION: Will be found useful in jaundice, gravel and female obstructions. Excellent results have been obtained by using the powdered root externally in cases of scrofulous tumors and ulcers.
METHOD: Decoction of 1 oz. to 1 pt. boiling water
DOSAGE: Wineglassful three or four times a day

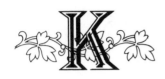

KIDNEY, SPLEEN, LIVER DISEASES,
AND URINARY COMPLAINTS

PLANT: Dodder   *Cuscuta epithymum*
WHERE FOUND: A parasitic plant found universally
PART USED: Herb
ACTION: Hepatic, laxative
DISSERTATION: Culpeper writes: "All Dodders are under Saturn. Tell me not of physicians crying up Epithymum, or that Dodder which grows upon Thyme ... he is a physician indeed, that hath wit enough to choose the Dodder according to the Nature of the disease and humour peccant. We confess Thyme is the hottest herb it usually grows upon; and therefore that which grows upon Thyme is hotter than that which grows upon cold herbs; for it draws nourishment from what it grows upon, as well as from the earth where its root is, and thus you see old Saturn is wise enough to have two strings to his bow."
METHOD: Infusion of 1 oz. of herb to 1 pt. boiling water
DOSAGE: Two to three teaspoonfuls twice daily

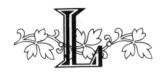

LARYNGITIS

PLANT: Pine Oils   *Abies sibirica, Pinus mugo, Pinus sylvestris*
WHERE FOUND: Europe and North America
PART USED: Oils
ACTION: Antiseptic, expectorant, inhalant, rubefacient
DISSERTATION: Above oils are widely used as inhalations for bronchitis and laryngitis. Also used in obstinate coughs and other chest conditions. Used as an ointment for eczema and other skin ailments.
METHOD: Apply Pumillo oil to the affected parts

LETHARGY

PLANT: Thyme, Wild or Mother of Thyme   *Thymus serpyllum*
WHERE FOUND: Europe, West Asia and North Africa
PART USED: Herb
ACTION: Antispasmodic, carminative, tonic
DISSERTATION: For convulsive coughs, whooping coughs, catarrh and sore throat.
METHOD: Infusion of 1 oz. herb to 1 pt. boiling water, sweetened with sugar or honey and made demulcent by Linseed or Acacia

DOSAGE: Tablespoonful doses frequently during the day

> Culpeper states: "It is under the dominion of Venus and under the sign of Aries and therefore chiefly appropriated to the head... If you make a vinegar of the herb and anoint the head with it, it presently stops the pains thereof. It is excellently good to be given either in phrenzy or lethargy, although they are two contrary diseases."

LIVER AND KIDNEY DISORDERS

PLANT: Dandelion *Taraxacum officinale*
WHERE FOUND: Everywhere; considered a pest and weed
PART USED: Root and leaves
ACTION: Aperient, diuretic, tonic
DISSERTATION: It is probably one of the most prescribed remedies on earth. It can be taken in any of many forms but it is claimed that its most beneficial action is best obtained in mixtures with other herbs. Chiefly used for liver and kidney disorders.
METHOD: The most pleasant way of taking this herb is in the form of a substitute for coffee. The roasted roots are ground and used as ordinary coffee, giving a beverage tasting much like the original article, and which certainly possesses most beneficial properties in cases of dyspepsia, gout, and rheumatism.

LIVER AND SPLEEN CONGESTION

PLANT: Bearsfoot, American   *Polymnia uvedalia*
WHERE FOUND: North America
PART USED: Root
ACTION: Anodyne, laxative, stimulant
DISSERTATION: It has been successfully used in congestion of the liver and spleen, enlarged womb, inflamed glands and dyspepsia. Used externally as a hair tonic or in the form of an ointment.
METHOD: Liquid extract
DOSAGE: 15 to 60 drops

LIVER AND SPLEEN OBSTRUCTIONS

PLANT: Hartstongue   *Scolopendrium vulgare*
WHERE FOUND: Found in the woodlands of Britain; also a garden plant
PART USED: Herb
ACTION: Diuretic, laxative, pectoral
DISSERTATION: Specially recommended for removing obstructions from the liver and spleen; also proven for removing gravelly deposits in the bladder.
METHOD: Decoction of 2 oz. to 1 pt. of water
DOSAGE: A wineglassful, as needed

Culpeper writes: "The distilled water is good for the passions of the heart, and gargled in the mouth will stay the hiccough, help the falling palate and stop the bleeding of the gums. It is a good remedy for the biting of serpents."

LIVER ENLARGEMENT

PLANT: Chicory   *Cichorium intybus*
WHERE FOUND: Popular garden plant in Great Britain and America; also grown commercially in Europe
PART USED: Root
ACTION: Diuretic, laxative, tonic
DISSERTATION: A decoction freely taken has proven effective in liver enlargement, gout and rheumatic complaints. This is the same root used in coffee mixtures, when roasted and ground.
METHOD: Decoction of 1 oz. root to 1 pt. boiling water
DOSAGE: Take freely

LOCKJAW

PLANT: White Pond Lily   *Nymphaea odorata*
WHERE FOUND: North America
PART USED: Root
ACTION: Antiseptic, astringent, demulcent
DISSERTATION: Valuable as a gargle for mouth and throat, and wash for sore eyes, ophthalmia and lockjaw. Good in bowel disorders. The powdered root combined with crushed linseed and powdered slippery elm makes a superb poultice. A decoction is used externally as an excellent lotion for bad legs and sores. Also good when used as an injection for leucorrhoea or gonorrhoea.
METHOD: Decoction of 1 oz. of root boiled for twenty minutes in 1 pt. of water
DOSAGE: Taken internally in wineglassful doses

LOOSE TEETH

PLANT: Pomegranate   *Punica granatum*
WHERE FOUND: Asia, the Caspian, the Persian Gulf, and the Mediterranean areas
PART USED: Fruit, rind of the fruit, bark of root, bark of stem
ACTION: Taenifuge
DISSERTATION: Joseph Miller states that Pomegranate is useful to strengthen the gums, fasten loose teeth, help the falling down of uvula and ulcers in the mouth and throat.

The art of making wine from pomegranates of which Solomon speaks is still practised in Persia.

A decoction of the bark of the root is considered a specific for removal of tapeworm.
METHOD: Decoction — 8 oz. of coarse bark of the root is put into a vessel and 3 pt. of cold water poured upon it. Boil for 1 hour, strain and boil it down until it measures 1 pint.
DOSAGE: Teacupful doses followed by a purgative. Repeat, if necessary, every 4 hours

LOOSENESS OF THE BOWELS

PLANT: Life Everlasting   *Antennaria dioica*
WHERE FOUND: America, Asia, Europe
PART USED: Herb
ACTION: Astringent
DISSERTATION: Taken internally as a styptic for looseness of the bowels. Also used as a gargle or an injection.

91

LUST, TO PROVOKE

PLANT: Prickly Asparagus   *Asparagus sativus*
WHERE FOUND: England
PART USED: Buds, root
ACTION: Aphrodisiac, cardiac, diuretic, laxative, sedative
DISSERTATION: According to Culpeper, "The decoction of the roots boiled in wine, and taken, is good to clear the sight, and being held in the mouth easeth the toothache; and being taken fasting several mornings together, stirreth up bodily lust in man or woman, whatever some have written to the contrary. The garden asparagus nourisheth more than the wild, yet hath it the same effects in all the aforementioned diseases."
METHOD: The freshly expressed juice is used or it can be made into a syrup
DOSAGE: Fresh juice — Taken in tablespoonful doses; Syrup — Taken in 1 to 2 tablespoonful doses

LUST, TO STOP

PLANT: Lady's Smock   *Cardamine pratensis*
WHERE FOUND: Great Britain, in low-lying places
PART USED: Herb and flowers
ACTION: Antiscorbutic, digestive, diuretic
DISSERTATION: It is regarded a powerful diuretic and recommended in convulsive disorders, nervous and hysteric cases, St. Vitus Dance and spasmodic asthma. An infusion assists both the veins and arteries.
METHOD: Infusion of 1 oz. in 1 pt. boiling water
DOSAGE: Taken in wineglassful doses

Culpeper says, "They are good for the scurvy, provoke urine, break the stone, and effectually warm a cold and weak stomach, restore lost appetite and help digestion."

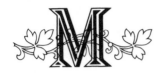

MALARIAL FEVERS

PLANT: Cashew Nut   *Anacardium occidentale*
WHERE FOUND: Native to West Indies but grows extensively
in the Levant and India
PART USED: Nut, bark
ACTION: Nutritive
DISSERTATION: The tree bark has proved efficient in certain
malarial fevers not yielding to treatment by quinine. The nut is
only edible after roasting. The fresh juice of the nut shell is
acrid, poisonous and corrosive, and the West Indian negroes use
it for removing warts and corns.

MALNUTRITION

PLANT: Dog-Rose   *Rosa canina*
WHERE FOUND: Almost universal
PART USED: Whole ripe fruit (hips)
ACTION: Corrects nutritional deficiencies
DISSERTATION: The hips (this applies to all rose species) if
eaten as found on the shrub are almost a complete food. They
contain invert sugar, citric acid, malic acid, and ascorbic acid
(vitamin C). Excellent food for infants and children who lack

proper food. Best when completely ground up 'meats' and seeds are sprinkled on food or even put into babies' bottles. Also made into a syrup and a conserve.

METHOD: Use in any of its many forms; that is, whole, ground or powdered

DOSAGE: Eat as much as you like, but eat it

MEMORY STRENGTHENER

PLANT: Melilot   *Melilotus officinalis*
WHERE FOUND: Grows freely in Great Britain and Europe
PART USED: Herb
ACTION: Aromatic, carminative, emollient
DISSERTATION: Taken internally to relieve flatulence. Externally, it is used as a poultice for aches and pains.

Culpeper states: "The head often washed with the distilled water of the herb and flowers or a lye made therewith, is effectual for those that have suddenly lost their senses, as also to strengthen the memory, comfort the head and brain, and to preserve them from pains and apoplexy."

MENTAL EXHAUSTION

PLANT: Ginseng   *Panax quinquefolium*
WHERE FOUND: China, Eastern U.S. and Canada
PART USED: Root
ACTION: Stimulant and tonic
DISSERTATION: Of value in any condition where nervous or

mental exhaustion is concerned. Accepted as being beneficial in loss of appetite, stomach and digestive affections.

METHOD: Powdered Root

DOSAGE: I5 grains immediately after meals

> The Chinese ascribe wonderful medicinal virtues to it. In fact, it was thought to be of such great service in so great a variety of complaints that it was given the botanical name "Panax," which means "all-healing" and is related to the word "Panacea."

MERRY, CHEERFUL, BLITHE SOUL, TO MAKE A

PLANT: Motherwort   *Leonurus cardiaca*

WHERE FOUND: Europe, and cultivated in Great Britain

PART USED: Herb

ACTION: Antispasmodic, emmenagogue, nervine, tonic

DISSERTATION: Culpeper writes: "There is no better herb to take melancholy vapours from the heart, to strengthen it, and make merry, cheerful, blithe soul than this herb."

METHOD: Powdered herb

DOSAGE: ½ to 1 dr.

> To many, Motherwort is known as a herb of life. There is an old saying, "Drink Motherwort and live to be a source of continuous astonishment and grief to waiting heirs."

MILK SECRETION OF NURSING MOTHERS, TO INCREASE

PLANT: Castor Oil Plant   *Ricinus communis*
WHERE FOUND: Native to India, but grown in gardens
PART USED: Leaves or oil from seeds
ACTION: Cathartic, purgative
DISSERTATION: Mild acting. Especially adapted for young children and pregnant women, in cases of constipation, colic and diarrhoea. Externally used for itch, ringworm and cutaneous complaints. The nauseous taste can be disguised by orange juice or lemon juice. The Canary Island child-bearing women use the fresh leaves applied to their breasts to increase the flow of milk.
METHOD: Oil of ricinus
DOSAGE: 60 to 240 min.

MORPHEW

PLANT: Alkanet   *Anchusa tinctoria*
WHERE FOUND: Montpellier
PART USED: Root
ACTION: Astringent, emollient
DISSERTATION: From Culpeper's Complete Herbal: "Dioscorides saith, it helps such as are bitten by venomous beasts, whether it be taken inwardly or applied to the wound; nay, he saith further, if any that hath newly eaten it do put spit into the mouth of a serpent, the serpent instantly dies. It stays the flux of the belly, kills worms, helps the fits of the mother. Its decoction made in wine, and drank, strengthens the back, and easeth the pains thereof. It helps bruises and falls, and is as gallant a remedy to drive out the smallpox and measles as any is: an ointment made of it is excellent for green wounds, pricks or thrusts."

MOSQUITO AND GNAT BITES

PLANT: Pennyroyal   *Mentha pulegium*
WHERE FOUND: Europe
PART USED: Herb, oil
ACTION: Carminative, diaphoretic, emmenagogue, stimulant
DISSERTATION: The oil is an excellent preventive application against the bites and stings of bees, gnats and mosquitoes.
     John Hill writes: "Mr. Boyle has left an account of its virtues against chin-cough; this is worth trying. The method of giving it is in the expressed juice, sweetened with sugar-candy, a spoonful for dose."
METHOD: An infusion, 1 oz. of herb in 1 pt. of boiling water.
DOSAGE: Warm teacupful doses, frequently

>   Gerard writes: "A garland of pennie-Royal made and worn about the head is of great force against the swimming of head and the pains and giddiness thereof."

MOTH REPELLENT FOR CLOTHES

PLANT: Wormwood   *Artemisia absinthium*
       Roman Wormwood   *Artemisia pontica*
       Common Wormwood   *Artemisia vulgaris*
WHERE FOUND: Worldwide
PART USED: Herb
ACTION: Anthelmintic, febrifuge, stomachic, tonic
DISSERTATION: Highly regarded for enfeebled digestion and debility.

Culpeper writes: "And why Roman seeing it grows familiarly in England? It may be so called, because it is good for a stinking breath which the Romans cannot be very free from, maintaining so many bad houses by authority of his Holiness." DOMESTIC USE: If wormwood is put where clothes are stored, it is said to keep moths away. It is also used in making Vermouth.

Culpeper states that Wormwood is good for preventing drunkenness. He quotes that when Saturn met with Venus and found her "drunk as a hog" Saturn said: "What, thou a fortune and be drunk? I'll give thee antipathetical cure; take my herb Wormwood and thou shalt never get a surfeit by drinking."

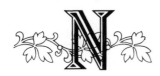

NERVE STIMULATING TONIC

PLANT: Kola   *Cola vera*
WHERE FOUND: Sierra Leone, North Ashanti, and also other tropical countries
PART USED: Seed
ACTION: Cardiac, diuretic, nerve stimulant, tonic
DISSERTATION: Because of the amount of Caffeine it contains, Kola acts as a good tonic. The African natives use it and it enables them to perform arduous tasks without food. Often prescribed for alcoholism.
METHOD: Powdered kola
DOSAGE: l5 to 45 gr.

NERVES

PLANT: Basil   *Ocimum basilicum*
WHERE FOUND: Planted widely in gardens, of Asiatic origin
PART USED: Herb
ACTION: Aromatic, carminative
DISSERTATION: Successfully used for centuries in mild nervous disorders. In South America it is used as a vermifuge.
METHOD: Make a hot tea — 1 teaspoonful to a pot of water

DOSAGE: Drink as tea, and also added to salads and soups.

NERVOUS DEBILITY, IRRITATION
AND HYSTERICAL AFFECTIONS

PLANT: Valerian   *Valeriana officinalis*
WHERE FOUND: Europe
PART USED: Rhizome
ACTION: Anodyne, antispasmodic, nervine
DISSERTATION: This herb may be used in all cases of nervous debility, irritation and hysterical affections. Also, it allays pain and promotes sleep. It is strongly nervine without any narcotic effects.
METHOD: Infusion of 1 oz. to 1 pt. of boiling water
DOSAGE: Wineglassful doses

NERVOUS PROSTRATION AND EXHAUSTION

PLANT: Oats   *Avena sativa*
WHERE FOUND: Widely distributed over Europe, Great Britain, North America and other countries
PART USED: Seeds or groats
ACTION: Antispasmodic, nerve tonic, stimulant
METHOD: Liquid extract is the form most used in treatment
DOSAGE: I0 to 30 drops

> Oats are known to be an important restorative in nervous prostration and exhaustion after all febrile diseases. It is also a tonic in spermatorrhoea and insomnia. It is claimed to exert a most beneficial action upon the heart muscles and on the urinary organs. Known to speedily relieve bladder and ureter spasms.

NEURALGIA

PLANT: Lady's Slippers   *Cypripedium pubescens*
WHERE FOUND: North America, Europe and Asia
PART USED: Rhizome
ACTION: Antispasmodic, nervine, tonic
DISSERTATION: Especially good for allaying neuralgic pains. Promotes sound slumber, relieves headache and female weakness. Given in hysteria and nervous disorders.
METHOD: Powdered root taken in water sweetened with honey
DOSAGE: 1 dr.

NEW ZEALAND CURE-ALL

PLANT: Kumarhou   *Pomaderris elliptica*
WHERE FOUND: North Island of New Zealand
PART USED: Herb
ACTION: Stimulant, tonic
DISSERTATION: The Maoris regard it as a general cure-all, especially for blood conditions. Claimed to be beneficial in cases of asthma, bronchitis and rheumatism. When combined with Vinca Rosea or alone, it is recommended for diabetes.
METHOD: Infusion of ½ oz. of herb to 1 pt. boiling water
DOSAGE: Wineglassful doses daily for at least 6 weeks

NOCTURNAL INCONTINENCE OF URINE

PLANT: Kava Kava   *Piper methysticum*
WHERE FOUND: South Sea Islands
PART USED: Root
ACTION: Diuretic, stimulant, tonic

DISSERTATION: Used in the east to strengthen the bladder and prevent the nocturnal incontinence of urine.
METHOD: Root
DOSAGE: 1 dr.

> The Natives ferment the root to make a liquor which causes a type of intoxication said to be quite distinct from that due to alcohol.

NOSEBLEED

PLANT: Fluellin   *Linaria elatine*
WHERE FOUND: Europe and Great Britain
PART USED: Herb
ACTION: Astringent
DISSERTATION: Recommended for internal bleeding, profuse menstruation and bleeding of the nose. It consolidates and strengthens.
METHOD: Infusion of 1 oz. herb to 1 pt. boiling water taken internally or applied to wounds
DOSAGE: Wineglassfuls as desired

> Culpeper describes it as a lunar herb and says: "The leaves bruised and applied with barley-meal to watering eyes that are hot and inflamed by defluxions from the head, helps them exceedingly."

104

OBESITY

PLANT: Samphire   *Crithmum maritimum*
WHERE FOUND: Grows along the seacoast in Europe
PART USED: Herb
ACTION: Diuretic
DISSERTATION: It is reputed to be an excellent treatment for obesity.
METHOD: Infusion of 1 oz. to 1 pt. boiling water
DOSAGE: Wineglassful doses taken freely

OBSTRUCTED PERSPIRATION

PLANT: Yarrow   *Achillea millefolium*
WHERE FOUND: Europe
PART USED: Herb
ACTION: Diaphoretic, stimulant, tonic
DISSERTATION: Considered valuable in obstructed perspiration, the commencement of fevers, and colds. It is said to freely open the pores and purifies the blood.
METHOD: Infusion of 1 oz. of herbs to 1 pt. of boiling water
DOSAGE: Wineglassful doses, drunk warm, with a teaspoonful of Composition Essence added to each dose. Combined with Elder flowers and Peppermint, it forms a speedy cure for influenza and colds.

OBSTRUCTION OF THE LIVER

PLANT: Tamarac   *Larix americana*
WHERE FOUND: North America
PART USED: Bark
ACTION: Alterative, diuretic, laxative
DISSERTATION: Highly esteemed in obstruction of the liver, jaundice, rheumatism, and skin disorders. Externally it is valuable in piles, menorrhagia, dysmenorrhoea.
METHOD: Decoction of bark, mixed with spearmint, juniper, horseradish, etc.
DOSAGE: Taken in wineglassful doses

OBSTRUCTIONS OF THE GALL

PLANT: Couchgrass or Dog's Grass   *Agropyron repens*
WHERE FOUND: Everywhere (Unhappily, as gardeners wail)
PART USED: Rhizome
ACTION: Aperient, demulcent, diuretic
METHOD: Infusion of 1 oz. to 1 pt. of boiling water
DOSAGE: Taken in wineglassful doses several times a day

Culpeper says that it "is the most medicinal of all the quick grasses. Being boiled and drunk it openeth obstructions of the liver and gall, and the stoppings of urine, and easeth the griping pains of the belly, and inflammations; wasteth the matter of the stone in the bladder, and the ulcers thereof also. The seed doth more powerfully expel urine, and stayeth laxes and vomiting.

OPHTHALMIA AND INDOLENT ULCERS

PLANT: Chickweed   *Stellaria media*
WHERE FOUND: Common weed almost everywhere
PART USED: Herb
ACTION: Demulcent, refrigerant
DISSERTATION: The fresh leaves have long been used, with great benefit, as a poultice for indolent ulcers and ophthalmia. An ointment has been used in treatment for cutaneous diseases. For scurvy and kidney conditions an infusion has proven a good remedy.
METHOD: Infusion of 1 oz. of herb to 1 pt. boiling water
DOSAGE: Wineglassful three or four times daily.

OPIATE

PLANT: Lettuce, Wild or Lettuce-opium   *Lactuca virosa*
WHERE FOUND: Central and Southern Europe
PART USED: Dried juice, leaves
ACTION: Anodyne, expectorant, sedative
DISSERTATION: Lactucarium is obtained by cutting the stem in sections and collecting the latex. Lettuce-opium is usually in angular fragments or quarters, curved on one side, indicating removal from a cup or saucer in which the milky juice has been collected and dried. Externally, it is dark reddish brown, internally, opaque and wax-like. Odour, resembling opium; taste very bitter.

Has been used when opium cannot be given. Most frequently it is used in the form of a syrup to sooth irritable coughs when such an agent is required. Used as an anodyne and hypnotic.
METHOD AND DOSAGE: Lactucarium — 5 to 15 gr.; Syrup — 2 dr.

ORDEAL IN WITCHCRAFT

PLANT: Sassy Bark   *Erythrophloeum guineense*
WHERE FOUND: Nyasaland, Sudan, West Coast of Africa
PART USED: Bark
ACTION: Astringent, laxative, narcotic
DISSERTATION: Used by the natives of West Africa as an ordeal in witchcraft. It contains toxic properties and should be handled with extreme caution.

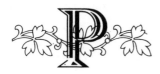

PAIN IN CANCEROUS GROWTHS

PLANT: Violet   *Viola odorata*
WHERE FOUND: Europe, Asia, Great Britain
PART USED: Leaves, flowers
ACTION: Antiseptic, expectorant
DISSERTATION: It has been recommended and used with benefit to allay pain in cancerous growths, some even say to cure cancer. In 1901 Lady Margaret Marsham of Maidstone, cured from cancer of the throat by infusion of Violet leaves published the recipe. The relief was almost immediate. In a week the external hard swelling had gone, and in a fortnight the cancer on the tonsil had disappeared. Pour a pint of boiling water on to a handful of fresh violet leaves and let stand for twelve hours. Strain when required. Apply to the affected part and cover with a piece of oilskin. Change the lint when dry or cold. Another report states that a gentleman aged 45 was cured of cancer by drinking 1 pint of infusion of violet leaves prepared from the dry leaves, and also by fomentation with the hot liquor. Or a poultice may be made and used in similar manner.

PAINFUL AND FREQUENT MICTURITION

PLANT: Eryngo   *Eryngium campestre*
WHERE FOUND: Found along the sea coast on sandy soil in
Europe and Great Britain
PART USED: Root
ACTION: Diaphoretic, diuretic, expectorant
DISSERTATION: Culpeper quotes an external use thus: "If the
roots be bruised, and boiled in old hog's grease, or salted lard,
and broken bones, thorns, etc., remaining in the flesh, they do
not only draw them forth, but heal up the place again, gathering
new flesh where it was consumed."

> **Women find it of benefit in uterine irritation, also bladder
> disease, painful and frequent micturition, with frequent
> ineffective attempts to empty the bladder.**

PAINS, INTERNAL AND EXTERNAL

PLANT: Cajuput   *Melaleuca leucadendron*
WHERE FOUND: East Indies
PART USED: Oil
ACTION: Antispasmodic, diaphoretic, stimulant
DISSERTATION: The natives of Molucca Islands, where the
tree grows, regard it very highly as a remedy for all sorts of
pains, internal and external. Made into a lotion it can be used
with benefit for rheumatic affections, toothache, neuralgia,
sprains and bruises. Internally taken on sugar in doses of 1 to 10
drops as a valuable diffusive stimulant in colics, spasms,

flatulence and hiccough.
METHOD: Oil of cajuput
DOSAGE: 1 to 3 min.

PARALYSIS, RHEUMATISM AND GOUT

PLANT: Bryony, Black   *Tamus communis*
WHERE FOUND: Europe
PART USED: Root
ACTION: Diuretic, rubefacient
DISSERTATION: Joseph Miller states, "A cataplasm of the root, with vinegar and cow-dung, helps the gout." Most significantly he adds, "It is but rarely used."
METHOD: The root is scraped and made into a pulp
DOSAGE: The resulting pulp is rubbed into the affected parts

PARASITICIDE AND INSECTICIDE

PLANT: Larkspur   *Delphinium consolida*
WHERE FOUND: European plant but naturalized wherever gardens are found
PART USED: Seeds
ACTION: Antibiotic
DISSERTATION: Used in spasmodic asthma and dropsy. A tincture of the seeds is effectively used as a parasiticide and insecticide. Old remedy for destroying lice and nits in the hair.
METHOD: Tincture of 1 oz. to 1 pt. dilute alcohol
DOSAGE: 10 drops and gradually increased

PAROXYSMAL ASTHMA

PLANT: Euphorbia   *Euphorbia hirta*
WHERE FOUND: Many tropical countries and India
PART USED: Herb
ACTION: Anti-asthmatic pectoral
DISSERTATION: Best known and used for the prompt relief it gives to sufferers of paroxysmal asthma.
METHOD: Infusion of 1 oz. to 1 pt. boiling water
DOSAGE: Tablespoonful doses as wanted

PELVIC FULLNESS

PLANT: Evening Primrose   *Oenothera biennis*
WHERE FOUND: America, but also grown in Europe and Great Britain
PART USED: Leaves and bark
ACTION: Astringent and sedative
DISSERTATION: Has been tested for various ailments and with considerable success in the treatment of gastro-intestinal disorders of a functional origin. Proven remedy for hepatic torpor, dyspepsia and female disorders connected with pelvic fullness. Of value in spasmodic asthma and whooping cough.
METHOD: Liquid extract
DOSAGE: ½ to 1 fluid dr.

PEPPER-UPPER

PLANT: Avens or Colewort   *Geum urbanum*
WHERE FOUND: Europe
PART USED: Root

ACTION: Astringent, febrifuge, stomachic, styptic, tonic
DISSERTATION: Claimed by some authorities to be the equal of Peruvian Bark in action in intermittent fevers. Has a pleasant taste. Has been used as an antiseptic remedy in cholera, morbus and dysentery. Also, in weakness of the stomach.
METHOD: 1 oz. powdered root to 1 pt. boiling water
DOSAGE: Wineglassful doses three or four times a day

PERCEPTION, TO IMPROVE

PLANT: Peyote or Mescal Buttons   *Lophophora Williamsi*
WHERE FOUND: Mexico and Texas
PART USED: Cut off tops are dried, resembling dried mushrooms
ACTION: Anodyne, emetic, febrifuge, hypnotic, narcotic
DISSERTATION: In Bailey's "Standard Cyclopedia of Horticulture" we read: "This plant is highly esteemed and even held in superstitious reverence by several tribes of Indians in the mountains of Mexico and in the United States, on account of its narcotic properties. It is said that it produces beautiful highly colored visions. Its taste is bitter and disagreeable, and it sometimes causes vomiting. The use of the drug is accompanied by the loss of a sense of time. Its effects have been compared to those of hasheesh (Cannabis indica), but that narcotic produces delusions of merriment while Lophophora causes a condition of ideal content followed by wakefulness. Several alkaloids have been separated from it, among them lophorine, anhalonine, and mezcaline."

It is said that the Indians of New Mexico and southwest United States "use the plant in manufacturing an intoxicating drink, also for breaking fevers" and that the tops cut off and dried are called mescal-buttons. These dried tops, which are often strung and sold in the markets of Mexico, look very much

113

like mushrooms and were mistaken for such by the early Spaniards. The Aztecs, who applied the name nanacatl to mushrooms in general, called this plant teonanacatl, which signifies "sacred mushroom."

PESTILENT FEVERS

PLANT: Barberry, Common *Berberis vulgaris*
WHERE FOUND: Europe
PART USED: Berries
ACTION: Diuretic, mild purgative, tonic
DISSERTATION: Useful in diarrhoea, dysentery, jaundice, intermittent fever and bronchitis.

In Thomas Green's "Universal Herbal" we read: "According to Prosper Alpinus, the Egyptians employ a diluted juice of the berries in ardent and pestilential fevers. Their method is to macerate them in about twelve times their quantity of water, and let them stand for about twenty-four hours, and then to add a little fennel seed. The liquor is then pressed out and strained, and sweetened with sugar, or syrup of citrons, roses, etc. and given plentifully as a drink."

PILES

PLANT: Pilewort *Ranunculus ficaria*
WHERE FOUND: Europe and Western Asia

PART USED: Herb
ACTION: Astringent
DISSERTATION: Pilewort, as its name indicates, is chiefly used for piles, for which it is almost a specific. Internally an infusion is used. Generally this is sufficient to cure most cases.
METHOD: Infusion of 1 oz. to 1 pt. boiling water
DOSAGE: Wineglassful doses

Sir James Sawyer, M.D., used the entire herb, macerated in boiling lard for 24 hours at a temperature of 100 deg. F., as an ointment for piles with good results. Applied locally twice daily.

PILES AND CHRONIC CONSTIPATION

PLANT: Cascara Sagrada   *Rhamnus purshiana*
WHERE FOUND: West coast of North America
PART USED: Bark
ACTION: Laxative and tonic
DISSERTATION: The bark must be more than a year old before it is used. Largely used for habitual constipation, dyspepsia and digestive complaints, and also for piles.
METHOD: Powdered bark
DOSAGE: 20 to 40 gr. at bedtime

PLAGUE

PLANT: Sage, Garden   *Salvia officinalis*

115

WHERE FOUND: Southern Europe
PART USED: Leaves
ACTION: Aromatic, astringent
DISSERTATION: Culpeper states: "The juice if drank with vinegar, is good for the plague. Gargles are made with sage, rosemary, honeysuckles, and plantain, boiled in wine or water, with some honey or alum added, to wash sore mouths and throats. Sage is boiled with other hot and comforting herbs, to bathe the body and the legs in the summer time, especially to warm cold joints or sinews, troubled with the palsy and cramp, and to comfort and strengthen the parts. It is recommended against the stitch, or pains in the side coming of wind, if the place be fomented warm with the decoction thereof in wine, and the herb also after boiling be laid warm thereunto."

PLAGUE AND PESTILENCE

PLANT: Juniper   *Juniperus communis*
WHERE FOUND: Widely distributed
PART USED: Berries and wood
ACTION: Carminative, diuretic, stimulant
DISSERTATION: Juniper Berries were used by the ancient herbalists of Greece and Arabia and by the Romans. The fifteenth and sixteenth century herbalists praised their use highly, their knowledge of their uses being culled to a large extent from the more ancient writers. The juice from the berries is recommended, as commonly are many herbs, against the bitings of vipers and against the plague and pestilence.

Parkinson writes: ". . . to procure safe and easy delivery unto woman with child, Mattheolus adviseth to take seven Juniper and seven Bayberries, half a dramme of Cassia lignea, and a dram of Cinamon, these being grossely bruised put them into the belly of a Turtle Dove to be roasted therewith, let it be basted with the fat of an Hen, whereof they are to eat every other evening . . ."

PLAGUE, FEVER OR HORROR

PLANT: Tormentilla   *Potentilla tormentilla*
WHERE FOUND: Europe
PART USED: Root and occasionally the herb
ACTION: Astringent, tonic
DISSERTATION: Parkinson writes, " . . . and so doth also the distilled water of the herbe and roote, rightly made and prepared, which is to steepe them in wine for a night and then distilled in Balneo marie; this water in this manner prepared taken with some Venice Treakle, and thereupon being presently laid to sweate, will certainly by God's helpe, expell any venome or poison, or the plague, or any fever or horror, or the shaking fit that happeneth . . ."

PLEURISY

PLANT: Crawley   *Corallorhiza odontorhiza*
WHERE FOUND: United States
PART USED: Rhizome (a parasitic leafless herb)
ACTION: Diaphoretic, febrifuge, sedative

DISSERTATION: Regarded of great value for the treatment of all fevers and pleurisy. It can be relied upon to produce free perspiration.
METHOD: Infusion of 1 oz. to 1 pt. boiling water
DOSAGE: Hot small cupfuls till results are produced

POISON

PLANT: Blessed Thistle   *Centaurea benedicta*
WHERE FOUND: Spain
PART USED: Leaves
ACTION: Alexipharmic, anthelmintic
DISSERTATION: Thomas Green states in his Universal Herbal: "This plant obtained the appelation *benedictus*, from its being supposed to possess extraordinary medical powers; for, exclusively of those qualities usually applied to bitters, it was thought to be a powerful alexipharmic, and capable of curing the plague and other malignant febrile disorders; it was also reputed to be good against worms, as well as against all sorts of poison. Simon Paulli declares, that it has no equal in consolidating putrid and stubborn ulcers, and even cancers. He relates the case of a woman, whose breasts were wasted by a cancer to the very ribs, and yet was cured by washing them with the distilled water of this plant, and sprinkling them with the powder of its leaves; and Arnoldus de Villa Nova relates, that he saw the putrid and hollow ulcers of a man, who had all the flesh of his legs consumed to the very bone, and who had tried all other medicines in vain, cured by the following recipe: Take the bruised leaves of this plant, and boil them with some generous wine, then add some melted hog's lard; let them boil a little more, and then put in some wheat flour, stirring it about all the while with a spatula, till it comes to the consistence of an ointment, which is to be laid warm upon the ulcers twice a day."

POLYPUS, HEMORRHAGES AND MUCOUS DISCHARGES

PLANT: Bistort   *Polygonum bistorta*
WHERE FOUND: Europe; likes shady places
PART USED: Root
ACTION: Astringent
DISSERTATION: Joseph Miller recommends the root for incontinence of urine.
METHOD: Decoction of 1 oz. to 1 pt. water
DOSAGE: Wineglassful as indicated

> Gerard states that the root boiled in wine "being holden in the mouth for a certain space and at sundry times, fasteneth loose teeth." He also says, "The juice of Bistort put into the nose prevaileth much against the disease called Polypus."

PREMATURE BALDNESS

PLANT: Rosemary   *Rosmarinus officinalis*
WHERE FOUND: Mediterranean regions
PART USED: Herb
ACTION: Astringent, diaphoretic, tonic
DISSERTATION: Used externally, an infusion combined with borax will prevent premature baldness and also makes an excellent hair wash.

"If a maid is curious as to her future she may obtain information by dipping a spray of Rosemary into a mixture of wine, rum, gin, vinegar and water in a vessel of ground glass. She is to observe this rite on the Eve of St. Magdelene in an upper

room in company with two other maids, and each must be less than 21 years old. Having fastened the sprigs to their bosoms and taken sips of the tonic — sips are quite enough — all three go to rest in the same bed without speaking. The dreams that follow will be prophetic."
METHOD: Infusion of 1 oz. herb to 1 pt. boiling water

PROLAPSE OF THE WOMB

PLANT: Madonna Lily   *Lilium candidum*
WHERE FOUND: Native to southern Europe, but grows widely in gardens
PART USED: Bulb
ACTION: Astringent, demulcent, mucilaginous
DISSERTATION: Combined with Life Root it is of value in treating prolapse of the womb and other female complaints.

Culpeper writes of Meadow Lily: "The root roasted, and mixed with a little Hog's grease, makes a gallant poultice to ripen and break plague-sores. The ointment is excellently good for swellings and will cure burnings and scaldings without a scar, and trimly deck a blank space with hair."
METHOD: Decoction of the bulb in milk taken internally
DOSAGE: Wineglassful doses

PSORIASIS, ECZEMA AND SCROFULOUS

PLANT: Chaulmoogra   *Taraktogenos kurzii*
WHERE FOUND: India and Malaysia
PART USED: Seeds from which the oil is pressed
ACTION: Dermatic, febrifuge, sedative
DISSERTATION: The oil from the seeds has been said to give good results as an internal and external remedy in scrofulous

and rheumatic skin affections. It has also proven itself a valuable remedy in stiffness of joints and skin eruptions such as psoriasis and eczema.

METHOD: Emulsion or ointment

DOSAGE: External ointment made of 1 part of oil to 4 of base. Internal, the oil is administered in the form of an emulsion with milk or ground almonds.

Chaulmoogra oil was once considered a specific in the treatment of leprosy.

PULMONARY COMPLAINTS

PLANT: Borage   *Borago officinalis*

WHERE FOUND: Throughout Europe; also grown in many gardens

PART USED: Leaves

ACTION: Demulcent, diuretic, emollient, refrigerant

DISSERTATION: Used in France for fevers and pulmonary disorders. Externally used as a poultice for inflammatory swellings. Dioscorides states that borage cheers the heart and helps dropping spirits.

METHOD: Infusion of 1 oz. leaves to 1 pt. boiling water

DOSAGE: Take in wineglassful doses

PULMONARY COMPLAINTS

PLANT: Beth Root   *Trillium erectum*
WHERE FOUND: North America
PART USED: Rhizome
ACTION: Alterative, astringent, pectoral, tonic
DISSERTATION: Useful in cases of internal bleeding, profuse menstruation and pulmonary complaints. Valuable in female disorders for the uterine organs. Was widely used by American Indians.
METHOD: One tablespoonful of powder in a pint of boiling water
DOSAGE: Take freely in wineglassful doses

PULMONIC CATARRH

PLANT: Pleurisy Root   *Asclepias tuberosa*
WHERE FOUND: North America
PART USED: Root
ACTION: Antispasmodic, carminative, cathartic, diaphoretic, expectorant, tonic
DISSERTATION: The name clearly suggests what time has made it famous for. Its greatest use is in pleurisy, in which condition it mitigates the pain and relieves the difficulty in breathing. Of immense value in all chest complaints and promotes a specific action on the lungs, assisting expectoration, subduing inflammation and exerting a generally mild tonic effect on the system. Highly recommended in pulmonic catarrh.
METHOD: Infusion of 1 teaspoon of the root to 1 cup of boiling water
DOSAGE: One or two cupfuls a day, cold

PUS IN BLADDER

PLANT: Corn Silk   *Zea mays*
WHERE FOUND: Wherever corn is grown
PART USED: Flower pistils of corn
ACTION: Demulcent, diuretic
DISSERTATION: Recommended as a valuable remedy in various urinary problems and bladder affections. Considered especially useful in purulent decomposition of urine in the bladder.
METHOD: Infusion of 2 oz. in 1 pt. boiling water
DOSAGE: Take freely

PYORRHOEA

PLANT: Witch Hazel   *Hamamelis virginiana*
WHERE FOUND: America
PART USED: Bark and leaves
ACTION: Astringent, sedative, tonic
DISSERTATION: Valuable in staying internal and external haemorrhages. Useful in piles. Recommended for pyorrhoea.
METHOD: For bleeding piles an ointment made by adding 1 part fluid bark extract to 9 parts simple ointment is used as a local application. For pyorrhoea massage the gums daily with Liquor Hamamelides.

QUINSY AND MUMPS

PLANT: Cudweed   *Gnaphalium uliginosum*
WHERE FOUND: Common in Great Britain; grows well in most barren places
PART USED: Herb
ACTION: Astringent
DISSERTATION: Regarded as an excellent remedy for quinsy.

Gerard writes: "Gnaphalium boiled in strong lee, cleanses the hair from nits and lice; also the herb being laid in ward-robes and presses keeps apparel from moths. The fume or smoke of the herb dried and taken with a funnel, being burned therein and received in such manner as we used to take tobacco that is with a crooked pipe made for the same purpose by the potter, prevaileth against the cough of the lungs, the great ache or pain of the head and cleanses the breast and inward parts."

According to Joseph Miller, Cudweed was so named because "It is given to cattle that have lost the ruminating faculty . . ."
METHOD: Infusion of 1 oz. to 1 pt. boiling water
DOSAGE: Wineglassful doses or as a gargle

Culpeper reports: "Pliny saith, the juice of the herb taken in wine and milk is a sovereign remedy against the mumps and quinsy ... whosoever shall so take it shall never be troubled with that disease again."

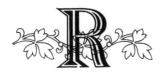

RASHES AND ITCHING

PLANT: Labrador Tea   *Ledum latifolium*
WHERE FOUND: North America
PART USED: Leaves
ACTION: Diuretic, expectorant, pectoral
DISSERTATION: A strong decoction has been recommended for external use as a remedy for itching and exanthematous skin diseases. Very useful in coughs, colds, bronchial and pulmonary complaints when taken internally as an infusion.
METHOD: Internal — Infusion of 1 oz. to 1 pt. boiling water; External — Use a stronger decoction.
DOSAGE: Decoction applied to affected parts; Infusion taken in wineglassful doses

RECTAL COMPLAINTS

PLANT: Horse Chestnut   *Aesculus hippocastanum*
WHERE FOUND: Native of North Asia
PART USED: Bark and fruit (seeds)
ACTION: Astringent, febrifuge, narcotic, tonic
DISSERTATION: The fruits have been successfully used for rectal complaints, backaches, piles, neuralgic and rheumatic

disorders and haemorrhoids. The bark is used in intermittent fevers. For ulcers the bark is used in external applications.

METHOD AND DOSAGE: Bark infusion of 1 oz. to 1 pt. boiling water, taken in teaspoonful doses four times a day. Fruits: Tincture 1 in 10 of proof spirit, 10 drops morning and night.

REDUCING AGENT

PLANT: Clivers   *Galium aparine*
WHERE FOUND: Europe and North America
PART USED: Herb
ACTION: Alterative, aperient, diuretic, tonic
DISSERTATION: Culpeper writes, "It is a good remedy in the spring, eaten in water-gruel, to cleanse the blood and strengthen the liver, thereby to keep the body in health, and fitting it for that change of season that is coming."

Considered of value in obstruction of urinary organs, suppression of urine and gravelly deposits. Said to act as a solvent of stone in the bladder.

METHOD: Infusion, hot or cold, of 1 oz. to 1 pt. water
DOSAGE: Frequent wineglassful doses

Gerard wrote, "Women do usually make a pottage of Clevers with a little mutton and oatmeale, to cause lankness and keep them from fatness."

RELAXATION OF UVULA

PLANT: Hollyhock, Common　　　　　　　　*Althaea rosea*
WHERE FOUND: In most gardens everywhere
PART USED: Flowers
ACTION: Demulcent, diuretic, emollient
DISSERTATION: Useful in chest complaints; similar in action to marshmallow.

　　　　Joseph Miller writes: "It is mostly used in gargles for the Swelling of the tonsils, and the relaxation of the Uvula; but it is not often met with in Prescriptions."

REMEDY AGAINST ANY DISEASE

PLANT: Golden Rod　　　　　　　　*Solidago virgaurea*
WHERE FOUND: Pernicious weed everywhere
PART USED: Leaves
ACTION: Aromatic, carminative, stimulant
DISSERTATION: Gerard, in addition to recommending Golden Rod against stone and pain in the kidneys, states: "It hath in times past been had in great estimation and regard . . . for in my remembrance I have known the dry herb which came from beyond the sea sold in Bucklerbury in London for half a crown an ounce. But since it was found in Hampstead Wood . . . no man will give half a crown for an hundredweight for it . . . yet it may be truly said of phantastical physitions who when they have an approved medicine and perfect remedy near home against any disease, yet not content therewith they will seek a new farther off and by that means many times hurt more than they help. Thus much have I spoken to bring those new fangled fellows back again to esteem better this admirable plant . . ."
METHOD: Infusion of 1 oz. leaves to 1 pt. boiling water
DOSAGE: Wineglassful doses frequently

REMOVING PROUD FLESH

PLANT: Raspberry   *Rubus idaeus*
WHERE FOUND: Temperate zone, cultivated berry plant
PART USED: Leaves and fruit
ACTION: Astringent, stimulant, tonic
DISSERTATION: An infusion is employed against diarrhoea and dysentery. Recommended for pregnant women as a tonic and to make parturition easy. Used also as a gargle for sore mouth and canker of the throat. Combined with Slippery Elm, the leaves make an excellent poultice for removing proud flesh and cleansing wounds.
METHOD: Infusion of 1 oz. leaves in 1 pt. boiling water
DOSAGE: Drink freely, nice and warm

RESTORES BURSTEN RUPTURES

PLANT: Rupturewort   *Herniaria glabra*
WHERE FOUND: England and the continent
PART USED: Herb
ACTION: Astringent, diuretic
DISSERTATION: Used in catarrhal affections of the bladder.
METHOD: Infusion of 1 oz. to 1 pt. boiling water
DOSAGE: Take freely

Gerard writes: "It is reported that being drunke it is singular good for Ruptures and that very many that have been bursten were restored to health by the use of this herbe also the powder hereof taken with wine . . . wasteth away the stone in the kidneys and expelleth them."

RETENTION OF URINE IN CHILDREN
AND KIDNEY DISEASE

PLANT: Clubmoss   *Lycopodium clavatum*
WHERE FOUND: Europe, Britain and most everywhere
PART USED: Plant and spores. The spores have a most unusual characteristic; they form a mobile powder which floats on water and does not get wet.
ACTION: Emollient and sedative
DISSERTATION: Best known taken internally for urinary disorders. Proven in treatment of spasmodic retention of urine in children, catarrhal cystitis and in chronic kidney diseases causing pain in kidneys, ureters and bladder, with rheumatic symptoms.
METHOD: Infusion of the moss, cut small — 1 oz. to 1 pt. boiling water
DOSAGE: Drink one cupful during the day, a large mouthful at a time

RINGWORM

PLANT: Jewel Weed   *Impatiens biflora*
WHERE FOUND: North America, East Indies
PART USED: Herb
ACTION: Aperient, diuretic
DISSERTATION: An excellent application for piles is made from fresh plants boiled with lard. The juice is reputed to cure ringworm and to remove warts and corns. In jaundice and dropsy the decoction is used.
METHOD: Decoction of 1 oz. to 1 pt. boiling water
DOSAGE: Wineglassful 3 to 4 times a day

RUPTURES AND BURSTINGS

PLANT: Five-Leaf-Grass   *Potentilla reptans*
WHERE FOUND: Common plant found widely scattered
PART USED: Herb, root
ACTION: Astringent, febrifuge
DISSERTATION: Found useful in diarrhoea and looseness of the bowels. Used externally as an astringent lotion.

Joseph Miller recommends the use of the root in the form of a gargle ''. . . for sore mouths and ulcerated gums and to fasten loose teeth.''
METHOD: Infusion of 1 oz. herb to 1 pt. boiling water
DOSAGE: Wineglassful doses

Gerard said, "The leaves are used among herbs appropriate for the same purpose to cure ruptures and burstings. The juice of the roots while they be young and tender is given to be drunk against the diseases of the liver and lungs and all poison."

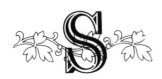

ST.VITUS DANCE

PLANT: Cohosh, Black   *Cimicifuga racemosa*
WHERE FOUND: North America and introduced into England
PART USED: Rhizome
ACTION: Alterative, astringent, emmenagogue, diuretic
DISSERTATION: Said to be a specific in St. Vitus Dance of children. Used as a remedy in rheumatism. Specially recommended for obstructed menses.
METHOD: Liquid extract
DOSAGE: 5 to 30 drops. DO NOT OVERDOSE for it produces nausea and vomiting.

SCARLET, TYPHOID AND INTERMITTENT FEVERS

PLANT: Eucalyptus   *Eucalyptus globulus*
WHERE FOUND: Native to Tasmania and Australia; cultivated in Southern Europe
PART USED: Leaves and oil distilled from them
ACTION: Antiseptic, antispasmodic, stimulant
DISSERTATION: In Australia it is a household remedy for many complaints. Has potent antiseptic qualities. Used as a local application in growths and wounds. Found beneficial in

ulcers. Also suggested for croup and spasmodic throat difficulties.

METHOD: Local application for ulcers, 1 oz. added to 1 pt. lukewarm water. For local injections, ½ oz. to 1 pt. lukewarm water. Internally, for scarlet fever, typhoid and intermittent fevers, the fluid extract is used and the oil is often applied freely to the body. Also used in this way for croup and spasmodic throat troubles.

SCIATIC PAINS

PLANT: Goutwort   *Aegopodium podagraria*
WHERE FOUND: A troublesome weed in Europe and the British Isles
PART USED: Herb
ACTION: Diuretic, sedative
DISSERTATION: Recommended internally for sciatic pains; also for aches in joints and gout. Used externally as a fomentation.

Culpeper states: "It is probable it took the name of Gout Herb from its peculiar virtues in healing the cold gout and sciatica as it hath been found by experience to be a most admirable remedy for these disorders. It is even affirmed, that the very carrying of it about in the pocket will defend the bearer from any attack of the aforesaid complaint."
METHOD: Liquid extract
DOSAGE: ½ to 1 dr.

SCIATICA OR ACHE IN THE HUCKLE BONE

PLANT: Poplar   *Populus tremuloides*

WHERE FOUND: North America and Europe
PART USED: Bark
ACTION: Diuretic, stimulant, tonic
DISSERTATION: Universal tonic, so it is described. Said to take the place of Peruvian Bark and Quinine.
METHOD: Liquid extract
DOSAGE: 1 dr.

Dioscorides wrote, "the barke to the weight of an ounce (or as other say, and that more truly a little more than a dram) is a good remedy for the sciatica or ache in the huckle bone."

SEDATIVE

PLANT: Asparagus   *Asparagus officinalis*
WHERE FOUND: Europe and Asia, but now cultivated everywhere
PART USED: Root
ACTION: Cardiac, diuretic, laxative, sedative
DISSERTATION: Long used because it is claimed to produce copious diuresis. It is recommended in dropsy, enlargement of the heart, and it has laxative qualities. This is the same asparagus used as the well known food delicacy.
METHOD: Freshly expressed juice
DOSAGE: Take in tablespoonful doses

SEDATIVE FOR THE NERVOUS SYSTEM

PLANT: Caroba   *Jacaranda caroba*
WHERE FOUND: South Africa and South America
PART USED: Leaves
ACTION: Alterative, diaphoretic, diuretic, sudorific
DISSERTATION: It appears to have a sedative effect on the nervous system but is rarely prescribed. It is used in epilepsy.
METHOD: Liquid extract
DOSAGE: 10 to 15 gr.

SEXUAL LASSITUDE AND RELIEF IN LABOUR PAINS

PLANT: Cotton Root   *Gossypium herbaceum*
WHERE FOUND: Asia Minor
PART USED: Bark of root
ACTION: Emmenagogue, oxytocic, parturient
METHOD: Infusion of 2 oz. to 1 pt. boiling water
DOSAGE: Wineglassful doses as applicable

Claimed to be safer and more effective in contracting the uterus than the widely known ergot. Long used in cases of difficult or obstructed menstruation. Especially recommended for use in sexual lassitude.

SEXUAL SEDATIVE

PLANT: Willow, Pussy   *Salix discolor*
WHERE FOUND: North America
PART USED: Bark, berries
ACTION: Anaphrodisiac, sexual sedative, tonic
DISSERTATION: Comes highly recommended and widely used in treatment of spermatorrhoea and nocturnal emissions. Relieves ovarian pain. Unrivalled in gangrene and indolent ulcers is a poultice made by simmering the powdered bark in cream.
METHOD: Infusion of 1 oz. bark to 1 pt. boiling water
DOSAGE: Wineglassful doses

SHINGLES, ECZEMA AND SCROFULA

PLANT: Walnut, English   *Juglans regia*
WHERE FOUND: Native to Persia but grown worldwide
PART USED: Bark, leaves
ACTION: Alterative, detergent, laxative
DISSERTATION: Has long been used in herpes or shingles, eczema and scrofula, taken as an infusion. Externally this is used as an application to skin eruptions and ulcers.
METHOD: Infusion of 1 oz. bark or leaves to 1 pt. boiling water
DOSAGE: Wineglassful doses as indicated

Waller states: The roots of the Walnut Tree laid bare and perforated, in the month of February yield a copious juice; it relieves chronic pains of the teeth, and even cures the pain of gout, and affords almost miraculous relief to those arising from stone and gravel both externally applied and internally drank ..."

SHORTNESS OF BREATH

PLANT: Nettle   *Urtica dioica*
WHERE FOUND: Universal
PART USED: Flowers, leaves, seeds
ACTION: Astringent, diuretic, nutritive, tonic
DISSERTATION: The seeds are used in coughs and shortness of breath. The herb makes a pleasant nutritional beer. It is also used as a medicine in nettle rash.

It is said that the Roman Nettle which thrives in England was originally planted there by Caesar's soldiers, who not having breeches thick enough to enable them to withstand the climate suffered much in the cold, raw fogs; so when their legs were numb they plucked nettles and gave those members such a scouring that they burned and smarted gloriously for the rest of the day.
METHOD: Infusion of 1 oz. of herb or seed to 1 pt. boiling water
DOSAGE: Wineglassful doses

SINGING IN THE EARS

PLANT: Savory, Summer   *Satureia hortensis*
WHERE FOUND: Garden plant grown throughout the world in gardens
PART USED: Herb
ACTION: Aromatic, carminative
DISSERTATION: Culpeper says of Summer Savory, "The juice heated with a little oil of roses, and dropped into the ears, easeth them of the noises and singing in them, and of deafness also. Outwardly applied with flour, in manner of a poultice, it giveth ease to the sciatica . . ."

138

SKIN CLEANSER

PLANT: Lovage or Tang Kui   *Levisticum officinale*
WHERE FOUND: Southern Europe
PART USED: Root
ACTION: Aromatic, carminative, diuretic, emmenagogue, stimulant, stomachic
DISSERTATION: Used in febrile affections, dysmenorrhoea and in stomach disorders.

Gerard writes: "The roots are very good for all inward diseases, driving away ventosities or windiness especially of the stomach. The seed thereof warmeth the stomach, helpeth digestion; wherefore the people of Gennes in times past did use it in their meats as we do pepper... The distilled water of Lovage clears the sight and puts away all spots, lentils, freckles and redness of the face, if they be often washed therewith."
METHOD: Liquid extract
DOSAGE: 5 to 30 min.

SKIN CLEANSER AND IMPROVER

PLANT: Elecampane   *Inula helenium*
WHERE FOUND: Parts of Europe and Asia; grown for botanical medicine use in Europe
PART USED: Root
ACTION: Alterative, diaphoretic, diuretic, expectorant
DISSERTATION: Usually mixed with other remedies for pulmonary troubles and coughs.
METHOD: Decoction of 1 oz. to 1 pt. boiling water
DOSAGE: Wineglassful doses as desired

SKIN DISEASES

PLANT: Boneset *Eupatorium perfoliatum*
WHERE FOUND: North America and Europe
PART USED: Herb
ACTION: Diaphoretic, expectorant, febrifuge, laxative, tonic
DISSERTATION: Will be found a certain remedy in cases of fever and influenza; also for catarrh and skin diseases. When used moderately it acts rapidly and effectively.
METHOD: An infusion of 1 oz. to 1 pt. boiling water
DOSAGE: Frequent wineglassfuls, hot to induce perspiration or cold as a tonic

SMALLPOX

PLANT: Pitcher Plant *Sarracenia purpurea*
WHERE FOUND: North America
PART USED: Root, leaves
ACTION: Diuretic, laxative, stomachic
DISSERTATION: At one time it achieved a great reputation as a prophylactic against small pox.
METHOD: Powdered root
DOSAGE: 10 to 20 gr.

140

SMALLPOX

PLANT: Henna   *Lawsonia alba*
WHERE FOUND: Arabia, Egypt, India, Persia
PART USED: Leaves
ACTION: Astringent
DISSERTATION: The natives of India and other Asiatic countries ascribe wonderful properties to this herb. They use it for smallpox, leprosy and headache. It is also used to dye the nails and hair.

SNUFF

PLANT: Galangal   *Alpinia officinarum*
WHERE FOUND: Island of Hainan and also along the coast of southeast China
PART USED: Rhizome
ACTION: Carminative, stimulant
DISSERTATION: The powdered rhizome is used as a snuff. The decoction is of great value in dyspepsia, for preventing fermentation and easing flatulence.
METHOD: Decoction of 1 oz. to 1 pt. boiling water
DOSAGE: Tablespoonful to wineglassful doses, as preferred. Powdered root is used in pinches as snuff.

SORE THROAT

PLANT: Cuckoopint   *Arum maculatum*
WHERE FOUND: Europe and the British Isles
PART USED: Root
ACTION: Diaphoretic, expectorant

DISSERTATION: A remedy internally and externally for sore throat.

Dioscorides states that the leaves are also used, but they must be eaten after they are dried and boiled. He further states that the root has a peculiar virtue against the gout "being laid on stamped with cow's dung."

METHOD: Powdered root

DOSAGE: 10 to 30 gr. NOTE: Large doses cause gastric inflammation and fatal results have been recorded.

Gerard writes: "Bears, after they have lain in their dens 40 days without any manner of sustenance but what they get with licking and sucking their own feet, do, as soon as they come forth, eat the herb Cuckoo-pint; through the windy nature thereof, the hungry gut is opened and made fit again to receive sustenance; for by abstaining from food for so long a time the gut is shrunk and drawn close together, that in a manner it is quite shut up."

SPERMATORRHOEA, AMENORRHOEA, DYSMENORRHOEA

PLANT: Cornsmut   *Ustilago maydis*
WHERE FOUND: Wherever corn is grown
PART USED: Fungus
ACTION: Emmenagogue, parturient
DISSERTATION: Has been used in labor, post-partum haemorrhages, as well as haemorrhages of lungs and bowels. Useful in menstrual derangements, spermatorrhoea, dysmenorrhoea and amenorrhoea.

142

METHOD: Liquid extract
DOSAGE: ½ to 2 dr.

SPITTING OF BLOOD

PLANT: Bugleweed   *Lycopus virginicus*
WHERE FOUND: Eastern North America
PART USED: Herb
ACTION: Aromatic, astringent, sedative, tranquilizer
DISSERTATION: Used in coughs. Has been used in enlargement of the thyroid gland. Said to be a positive remedy in haemoptysis. Promotes digestion and increases the appetite.
METHOD: Infusion of 1 oz. to 1 pt. boiling water
DOSAGE: Take glassfuls frequently

SPLEEN AND LIVER AFFECTIONS

PLANT: Cup-Plant   *Silphium perfoliatum*
WHERE FOUND: India
PART USED: Rhizome
ACTION: Alterative, diaphoretic, tonic
DISSERTATION: Long known as a general restorative. Years have established its value in spleen and liver affections; also useful in fevers.
METHOD: Decoction of powdered root
DOSAGE: Wineglassful doses at intervals

SPONGY AND BLEEDING GUMS

PLANT: Rhatany   *Krameria triandra*
WHERE FOUND: Bolivia and Peru
PART USED: Root
ACTION: Astringent, tonic
DISSERTATION: It is useful as an application to spongy and bleeding gums. Used internally with good results in passive haemorrhages, mucous discharges and menstrual complaints.
METHOD: Extr. Kramer. B.P.C.
DOSAGE: 5 to 15 gr.

SPONGY GUMS AND SORE THROAT

PLANT: Catechu, Black   *Acacia catechu*
WHERE FOUND: India and Burma
PART USED: Extract from leaves and young shoots
ACTION: Astringent
DISSERTATION: Used as a local application in relaxed sore throat and sponginess of gums. Useful for arresting excessive mucous discharges and for checking haemorrhages.
METHOD: Powdered Catechu
DOSAGE: 5 to 15 gr.

STERILITY

PLANT: Leek   *Allium porrum*
WHERE FOUND: Common garden vegetable
PART USED: Bulb, juice
ACTION: Diuretic, stimulant
DISSERTATION: The Leek has long been esteemed in

barrenness, as has Speedwell. Highly esteemed by the French and Germans. Constipation must be avoided.

METHOD: Expressed juice

DOSAGE: Teaspoonful doses

Hill states "An infusion of the roots boiled into a syrup with honey, is a good medicine in coughs, asthma and disorders of the breast and lungs."

STIFF NECK

PLANT: Woollen or Cotton Thistle *Carlina vulgaris*

WHERE FOUND: Mediterranean regions

PART USED: Root, leaves

ACTION: Antiscorbutic, nervine

DISSERTATION: Matthew Robinson wrote in his herbal, "Dioscorides and Pliny write, that the leaves and roots taken in drink, cure stiff neck. Galen says that the roots and leaves are good for such persons that have their bodies drawn together by spasm or convulsion, or other infirmities; as the rickets in children, a disease that hinders their growth, by binding their nerves, ligaments, etc. It is good also in nervous complaints."

STIMULANT

PLANT: Buchu *Barosma betulina*

WHERE FOUND: South Africa; especially in the Cape area

145

PART USED: Leaves
ACTION: Diaphoretic, diuretic, stimulant, tonic
DISSERTATION: It exorts a direct effect on the urinary organs, with much benefit. Also useful in gravel, inflammation and catarrh of the bladder.
METHOD: An infusion of 1 oz. of leaves to 1 pt. boiling water
DOSAGE: Wineglassful doses three or four times a day

STIMULANT AND HEAT PRODUCER

PLANT: Cayenne   *Capsicum frutescens*
WHERE FOUND: East Indies, India, Japan, Africa and tropical America
PART USED: Fruit
ACTION: Carminative, rubefacient, stimulant, tonic
DISSERTATION: Considered the purest and most positive stimulant in the herbal materia medica.
METHOD: Capsicum powder
DOSAGE: ½ to 2 gr.

It does produce natural heat and will equalize or increase circulation. Said to ward off colds if used at the first signs. Considered a very important remedy in herbal practice.

STINGS BY BEES AND WASPS

PLANT: Blue Mallow   *Malva sylvestris*

WHERE FOUND: Europe and the British Isles
PART USED: Herb, flowers
ACTION: Demulcent, mucilaginous, pectoral
DISSERTATION: The infusion is a popular remedy for coughs, colds and bronchial complaints. A fomentation is used to soften abscesses.

Joseph Miller said, "A cataplasm of the leaves applied to the place, stung by bees or wasps, eases the smart."
METHOD: Infusion for coughs, etc.: 1 oz. to 1 pt. boiling water
DOSAGE: Wineglassful three times a day

STINKING BREATH

PLANT: Rest Harrow   *Ononis spinosa*
WHERE FOUND: Mediterranean areas
PART USED: Root
ACTION: Diuretic
DISSERTATION: Parkinson writes, "Four pounds of the roots first sliced small and afterwards steeped in a gallon of Canary Wine . . . and put into a stone pot close stopped . . . and so set to boyle in a Balneo Marie for 24 hours is as daintie a medicine for tender stomachs as any the daintiest Lady in the land can desire to take . . ."

Also Parkinson: "It is recorded that in former times the young shoots and tender stalks before they become prickly were pickled up to bee eaten as a meate or sauce, wonderfully commended against a stinking breath, and to take away the smell of wine in them that had drunk too much."

STONES AND GRAVEL IN THE BLADDER

PLANT: Hydrangea   *Hydrangea arborescens*
WHERE FOUND: Native to the United States, but grown widely
PART USED: Root
ACTION: Cathartic, diuretic, nephritic
DISSERTATION: Long recognized as a valuable remedy for the removal of stone and gravel in the bladder. Its best known use is in the prevention of any gravelly deposits.
METHOD: Infusion of 1 oz. root in 1 pt. boiling water
DOSAGE: Take hot or cold in wineglassful doses

STONES IN KIDNEYS AND BLADDER

PLANT: Birch, European   *Betula alba*
WHERE FOUND: Europe, but similar tree in North America
PART USED: Bark and leaves
ACTION: Astringent, bitter
DISSERTATION: Most of the old herbalists claim that "the juice of the leaves when young or the water distilled from them, or the water from the tree after it has been bored with an auger, being taken for some days together, breaks the stone in the kidneys and bladder."
METHOD: Infusion of 1 oz. leaves to 1 pt. boiling water
DOSAGE: Small wineglassfuls as required

STRANGE SIGHTS AND FANCIES – HALLUCINATIONS

PLANT: Bugle   *Ajuga reptans*
WHERE FOUND: Throughout Europe

PART USED: Herb
ACTION: Aromatic, astringent
METHOD: Infusion of 1 oz. to 1 pt. boiling water
DOSAGE: A wineglassful taken frequently

Culpeper states, "Many times such as give themselves to drinking are troubled by strange fancies, strange sights in the night and some with voices ... Those I have known cured by taking only two spoonfuls of the syrup of this herb after supper two hours, when you go to bed ..."

STY

PLANT: Witch Hazel   *Hamamelis virginiana*
WHERE FOUND: Native to the United States
PART USED: Bark, leaves
ACTION: Astringent, sedative, tonic
DISSERTATION: Most valuable in checking internal and external haemorrhages; also for the treatment of piles. A decoction made from the bark of leaves makes an excellent injection for bleeding piles. An ointment made by adding 1 part fluid extract bark to 9 parts simple ointment is also used as a local application. For treatment of sty in the eye, careful application of the ointment has proven effective.
METHOD: Ointment
DOSAGE: Local application

STYPTIC AND PURGATIVE

PLANT: Rhubarb   *Rheum palmatum*
   (Not Common Rhubarb which is known as Rhaponticum)
WHERE FOUND: China
PART USED: Rhizome
ACTION: Astringent, aperient, stomachic, tonic
DISSERTATION: In small doses the powder will stop diarrhoea; in large doses it is a simple and safe purgative. It is said to be one of the most valuable remedies that "we possess."
      Externally it is used as an astringent or styptic to stop bleeding.
METHOD: Tincture or powder
DOSAGE: Sprinkle powder lightly over bleeding area

SUPPRESSED MENSTRUATION

PLANT: Life Root   *Senecio aureus*
WHERE FOUND: America and Europe
PART USED: Herb, rhizome
ACTION: Astringent, diuretic, emmenagogue, pectoral, tonic
DISSERTATION: A highly valued botanical deserving of careful study. It is regarded by many authorities as a specific for suppressed menstruation. It is also of value in gravel, stone and diarrhoea.
      For pulmonary complaints — 1 teaspoonful of the fluid extract should be taken in sweetened water or combined with other pectorals.
METHOD: For suppressed menstruation — ½ oz. of powder or fluid extract in 1 pt. water
DOSAGE: Wineglassful doses four times a day till desired results are obtained

SUPPURATING TUMOURS

PLANT: Onion   *Allium cepa*
WHERE FOUND: Universal
PART USED: Bulb
ACTION: Diuretic, expectorant
DISSERTATION: Roasted onion as a poultice for suppurating tumours. The same treatment is used for earache. A syrup made from the juice makes a beneficial cough medicine. For gravel and dropsical affections onions are macerated in Gin to make a tincture.

SUPPURATION PREVENTIVE

PLANT: Marigold or Pot Marigold   *Calendula officinalis*
WHERE FOUND: Mediterranean areas; widely grown in gardens
PART USED: Petals, herb
ACTION: Diaphoretic, stimulant
DISSERTATION: Generally used as a local remedy. Taken internally it assists the local action and prevents suppuration. Used for chronic ulcers and varicose veins.

Gerard writes "Fuchius writeth that if the mouth be washed with the juice it helpeth the tooth-ache."

He also states: "The leaves of the flowers are dried and kept throughout Dutchland against winter to put in broths, in Physical potions, and for divers other purposes, in such quantity that in some grocers or spice sellers houses are to be found barrels filled with them and retailed by the penny more or less, insomuch that no broths are well made without dried Marigolds."
METHOD: Infusion of 1 oz. of herbs and petals to 1 pt. boiling water
DOSAGE: Tablespoonful to wineglassful doses, and also as an application for external purposes

151

SWELLING OF THE TESTICLES

PLANT: Rue or Herb of Grace   *Ruta graveolens*
WHERE FOUND: Southern Europe, but cultivated worldwide
PART USED: Herb
ACTION: Antispasmodic, carminative, emmenagogue, nervine, stimulant
DISSERTATION: Recommended in nervous complaints, flatulence, colic, epilepsy and hysteria. It can cause abortion.

Dioscorides states that "a twelve pennyweight of the seed drunk in wine is a counterpoison of serpents, the stinging of scorpions, bees, hornets and wasps; and it is reported that if a man be anointed with the juice of the Rue, these will not hurt him; and that the serpent is driven away at the smell thereof when it is burned; insomuch that when the weasel is to fight with the serpent she armeth herself by eating Rue, against the might of the serpent."
METHOD: Infusion of 1 oz. to 1 pt. boiling water
DOSAGE: Teacupful doses as required

SYPHILIS

PLANT: Sarsaparilla, Jamaica   *Smilax ornata*
WHERE FOUND: Central America
PART USED: Root
ACTION: Alterative
DISSERTATION: Has been found that it contains active alterative qualities that still cause it to be held in high esteem as a general purifier of the blood. Best results are found in conjunction with other remedies, such as Sassafras and Burdock.
METHOD: Powdered Root
DOSAGE: ¼ to 1 dr.

This root was introduced by the Spaniards back in 1563 as a sure cure for Syphilis. It has been thoroughly tested since then and experience has demonstrated that it is not an absolute specific.

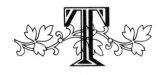

TAPEWORM

PLANT: Embelia   *Embelia ribes*
WHERE FOUND: India
PART USED: Fruit
ACTION: Carminative, diuretic, taenicide
DISSERTATION: The natives of the East Indies use it in dyspepsia and rheumatic affections. It is best known and mainly used for its ability to expel tapeworms.
METHOD: The seed (fruit) when powdered is used mixed with milk
DOSAGE: Take 1 to 3 tsps. mixed with milk, on an empty stomach, followed by a purgative

TARTAROUS INCRUSTATIONS ON THE TEETH

PLANT: Strawberry   *Fragaria vesca*
WHERE FOUND: Europe
PART USED: Fruit, leaves and root
ACTION: Astringent, diuretic, nervine
DISSERTATION: Thomas Green states in his Universal Herbal: "They promote perspiration, impart a violet scent to the urine, and dissolve the tartarous incrustations upon the teeth. Persons

155

afflicted with the gout or stone, have found great relief by using them profusely. Linneus informs us that by eating plentifully of them every day, he kept himself almost free from the gout. Hoffman affirms, that he has known consumptive people cured by them. The bark of the root, like that of the tormentil, and the rest of its congener, is astringent. The leaves, says Meyrick, are cooling and diuretic: an infusion of them is good in the strangury; and when made strong, in the jaundice; when dried and reduced to powder, they are astringent, and useful in fluxes of the bowels; and a strong decoction of them sweetened with honey, is a good gargle for sore throats. It would be unpardonable not to inform our fair readers, that they have likewise the credit of being a cosmetic, or beautifier of the skin."

TETTERS

PLANT: Holy Thistle   *Cnicus benedictus*
WHERE FOUND: Mediterranean area, Caucasus and southern United States
PART USED: Herb
ACTION: Diaphoretic, emmenogogue, tonic
DISSERTATION: Very useful for intermittent fevers, breaking up colds, loss of appetite, and dyspepsia.
METHOD: 1 oz. herb to 1 pt. boiling water
DOSAGE: Warm wineglassful doses as desired

Culpeper says, "It strengthens the attractive faculty in man and clarifies the blood, because the one is ruled by Mars. The continually drinking the decoction of it helps red faces, tetters, and ringworms, because Mars causeth them."

THROAT AFFECTIONS, HOARSENESS, INFLAMMATORY DISEASES

PLANT: Black Currant   *Ribes nigrum*
WHERE FOUND: Grown widely in gardens; highly esteemed for jams and jellies
PART USED: Leaves, fruit
ACTION: Leaves are detergent, diuretic, refrigerant
DISSERTATION: Very useful in febrile and inflammatory diseases, in hoarseness and affections of the throat
METHOD: Infusion of 1 oz. in 1 pint of boiling water
DOSAGE: Take in teacupful doses

THROAT RELAXER

PLANT: Oak Galls   *Quercus infectoria*
WHERE FOUND: Greece, Syria and Turkey
PART USED: The excrescence or the gall
ACTION: Astringent
DISSERTATION: Used as a gargle it will sooth and relax the throat. Also used in cholera, diarrhoea, dysentry and passive hemmorrhages. The infusion may be used as an injection in leucorrhoea
METHOD: Infusion of 1 oz. herb to 1 pt. boiling water
DOSAGE: Wineglassful, as gargle

THRUSH

PLANT: Myrrh   *Commiphora molmol*
WHERE FOUND: Arabia and North East Africa
PART USED: Oleo-gum-resin
ACTION: Healing antiseptic, stimulant, tonic

DISSERTATION: A valuable and deservedly popular medicine. The tincture is used in thrush, inflammatory sore throat, ulcers, bad legs, and other complaints. It makes an excellent wash for ulcerated mouth and tongue.
METHOD: Tincture of Myrrh B.P.C.
DOSAGE: 30 to 60 min.

THRUSH (LITTLE ULCERS IN THE MOUTH)

PLANT: Arsesmart   *Polygonum hydropiper*
WHERE FOUND: Europe, but naturalized everywhere
PART USED: Herb, leaves
ACTION: Emmenagogue, diuretic, stimulant
DISSERTATION: Thomas Green states in his Universal Herbal: "From its hot acrid taste, it has the names of Hydropiper, Water Pepper, Persicaria; and another still more significant appelation, which has now become so offensive in the ears of modern refinement, that one would think the present polite generation were in no instance troubled with that ignoble part from which this indelicate name is derived. Withering observes, that the whole plant has an exceeding hot biting taste. It cures those little ulcers in the mouth commonly called the thrush; and the distilled water, drank to the quantity of a pint or more in a day, has been found serviceable in the gravel and stone. It is a diuretic of considerable efficacy, and has frequently been administered with success in the jaundice, and the beginning of dropsies. The express juice of the fresh-gathered plant appears to be the best preparation of it, and may be taken with safety to the amount of two or three ounces for a dose."
METHOD: Infusion of 1 oz. of leaves in 1 pt. of cold water
DOSAGE: Wineglassful doses as wanted

THYROID GLAND, TO IMPROVE FUNCTION OF

PLANT: Bladderwrack   *Fucus vesiculosus*
WHERE FOUND: Off the British coasts and other coasts
PART USED: Whole Plant
ACTION: Alterative, deobstruent, diuretic
DISSERTATION: Potter states that it has been used with success in obesity. Said to have the ability to clear away obstructions by opening the natural passages of the body. Has been used for centuries as an animal food, especially during the winter. Said to keep animals in excellent health.

It was employed for making iodine of benefit for fatty degeneration of the heart, stomach and intestinal conditions, difficult breathing and dyspnea. The drug acts on the thyroid gland by furnishing iodine and thus improves its functions. Has a mouldy, salty, but not unpleasant flavor.

TIRED FEET AND WEARINESS

PLANT: Lady's Bedstraw   *Galium verum*
WHERE FOUND: Europe and naturalized in North America
PART USED: Herb
ACTION: Alterative, diuretic
DISSERTATION: Has been used for gravel, stone, urinary disease, epilepsy and hysterical complaints.

Parkinson writes: " ... these sorts with white flowers have been thought unprofitable, and of no use, but Clausius saith, the poor women in Austria, Hungaria and other places in Germany that gather herbs and roots for their uses that need them, bringing them to the market to sell ... by their experience found it good for the sinews arteries and joints, to bath them therewith both to take away their weariness and weakness in them, and to comfort and strengthen them also after travail,

cold or pains."
METHOD: Infusion of 1 oz. herb to 1 pt. boiling water
DOSAGE: Wineglass doses several times a day

> Joseph Miller says: "Some commend a decoction of it for the gout; and a bath made of it is very refreshing to wash the feet of persons tired with overwalking."

TO MAKE GUESTS MERRIER

PLANT: Vervain   *Verbena officinalis*
WHERE FOUND: Central America and Europe
PART USED: Herb
ACTION: Emetic, nervine, sudorfic, tonic
DISSERTATION: Pliny is claimed to have said, and confirmed by Dioscorides, that "If the dining room be sprinkled with water in which the herb hath been steeped the guests will be merrier."

Joseph Miller states: "The whole herb is used being accounted cephalic and good against diseases from cold and phlegmatic causes; it opens obstructions of the Liver and Spleen, helps the Jaundice and Gout, and applied outwardly is reckon'd vulnerary and good for sore watery inflamed eyes."

TONIC

PLANT: Peruvian Bark   *Cinchona officinalis*
WHERE FOUND: South America
PART USED: Bark
ACTION: Astringent, febrifuge, tonic

160

DISSERTATION: Claimed in some respects to be one of the most remarkable remedies ever discovered. Must be properly used — not abused. For years there has been a strong tendency to overdose and this undoes the many benefits that might accrue from the use of this fine herbal remedy. Used for a tonic and nervous dyspepsia, dyspepsia due to lack of hydrochloric acid in the stomach, bowel pains due to accumulation of gas, intermittent fevers, malaria, ringing in the ears, catarrh, colds and complaints brought on by colds, liver and spleen dysfunction, jaundice, gastro duodenal catarrh, painful periods, asthma worsened by bad weather, influenza, pains in limbs and joints, debility, nervous exhaustion, and last, but not least, it is wonderful for rebuilding the body after an exhaustive illness.
METHOD: Tincture
DOSAGE: Take 5 to 10 drops in warm water three times a day

TOOTHACHE

PLANT: Pellitory of Spain　　　　　　　*Anthemis pyrethrum*
WHERE FOUND: Southern Europe
PART USED: Root
ACTION: Pungent, stimulant
DISSERTATION: Thomas Green states in his Universal Herbal: "When chewed, it excites a glowing heat, with a discharge of saliva, which relieves toothache and rheumatic affections of the face: it is also recommended in lethargic complaints and paralyses of the tongue. Lewis says, the roots having a hot pungent taste when chewed in the mouth, by stimulating the salival glands, promote a flow of viscis humours from the head and the adjacent parts, and frequently by this means relieve the toothache, headache, lethargy, and palsy of the tongue. It is also successfully given in small doses for paralytic and rheumatic complaints. In palsies, its stimulation alone will sometimes restore the voice."

161

TRANQUILITY

PLANT: Asafetida or Devil's Dung   *Ferula foetida*
WHERE FOUND: Afghanistan, Persia
PART USED: Oleo-gum-resin
ACTION: Antispasmodic, expectorant, nervine, stimulant
METHOD: A pinch of the powdered gum-resin in a glass of hot water
DOSAGE: Taken hot in wineglassful doses before bedtime and before meals

---

Employed as a nervous sedative for its tranquilizing effect. Useful in neurasthenia, hysterical disorders, bronchitis, asthma, St. Vitus Dance, infantile convulsions, croup, flatulence, colic and gastric irritation. Due to the plant's strong garlic-like odor and harsh bitter garlic-like taste, it is often taken in capsule form.

TREMBLING OF THE HEART

PLANT: Dodder   *Cuscuta europaea*
WHERE FOUND: British heaths
PART USED: Herb
ACTION: Aperient, deobstruent, hepatic
DISSERTATION: Opens the obstructions of the liver, and is good in jaundice and for the spleen.

Culpeper states: "This is accounted the most effectual for melancholy diseases, and to purge black or burnt choler, which is the cause of many diseases of the head and brain, as also for the trembling of the heart, faintings, and swoonings. It is helpful in all diseases and griefs of the spleen, and melancholy that arises from the windiness of the hypocondria. It purgeth also the reins or kidneys by urine; it openeth obstructions of the gall, whereby it profiteth them that have the jaundice; as also the leaves the spleen; purging the veins of choleric and phlegmatic humours, and helpeth children in agues, a little worm seed being added thereto."

METHOD: Decoction of 1 oz. to 1½ pts. of water

DOSAGE: Wineglassful doses as required

TREMORS OF THE LIMBS

PLANT: Lily of the Valley   *Convallaria majalis*

WHERE FOUND: Common garden flower

PART USED: Flower

ACTION: Cardiac, diuretic, stimulant, tonic

DISSERTATION: "An infusion of the flowers constantly taken instead of tea is an excellent remedy for nervous headaches, trembling of the limbs and other similar complaints."

TRUE TONIC, SUPER EXCELLENT

PLANT: Gentian   *Gentiana lutea*

WHERE FOUND: Mountain areas of Europe, Asia, elsewhere

PART USED: Root

ACTION: Tonic

DISSERTATION: Rated and recognized as the most valuable and popular tonic medicine in the entire botanical kingdom. Bitter but without biting, it is the safest of all tonic herbs. Benefits the digestion and aids general debility, female weakness and hysteria.

    Culpeper writes: "They are under the dominion of Mars,

and one of the principal herbs he is ruler of. They resist putrefactions, poison, and a more sure remedy cannot be found to prevent the pestilence than it is."
METHOD: Powdered Root
DOSAGE: 10 to 30 gr.

> Parkinson writes of the esteem in which this plant was held by the Germans who made with it a treacle used as a counter-poison " ... made of Gentian, Aristolochia, Bayberries and other things ..."

TUMOURS, ABSCESSES, GATHERINGS

PLANT: Ground Ivy   *Glechoma hederacea*
WHERE FOUND: Grows wild and is common to Europe and Britain
PART USED: Herb
ACTION; Astringent, diuretic, pectoral, stimulant, tonic
DISSERTATION: Has wide use for many complaints. Has antiscorbutic qualities. Useful for indigestion and kidney diseases. When made into a poultice, mixed with yarrow and chamomile flowers, it is excellent for tumours, abscesses and gatherings.

Gerard recommends: "Ground Ivy, and Daisies, of each a like quantity, stamped and strained, and a little sugar and rose water put thereto, and dropped with a feather into the eyes, taketh away all manner of inflammation, spots, webs, itch, smarting, or any grief whatsoever ... "

Parkinson says of Ground Ivy: "The country people do much use it and tune it up with their drink, not only for the especially good virtues therein, but for that it will help also to clear their drink ... "
METHOD: Infusion of 1 oz. herb to 1 pt. boiling water
DOSAGE: Wineglassful twice a day

TYPHUS FEVER AND SKIN DISEASES

PLANT: Contrayerva   *Dorstenia contrayerva*
WHERE FOUND: West Indies, Mexico, Peru
PART USED: Rhizome
ACTION: Diaphoretic, stimulant
DISSERTATION: Its many excellent qualities make it an excellent remedy in typhus fever, dysentery and skin diseases.
METHOD: Infusion of 1 oz. in 1 pt. boiling water
DOSAGE: Wineglassful as needed.

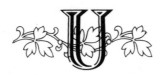

ULCEROUS WOUNDS, ASTHMA, HAY FEVER

PLANT: Comfrey   *Symphytum officinale*
WHERE FOUND: Russia, Great Britain, and transplanted anywhere
PART USED: Leaves and roots (whole plant)
DISSERTATION: One of the highest rated plants in the modern herbal calendar. It appears well worth trying in any complaint that does not readily yield to other treatments.
METHOD: Used as a poultice, eaten like lettuce, or the leaves dried and made into a tea by infusion. Decoction of the root: 1 oz. of crushed root in 1 qt. of water
DOSAGE: As tea, can be drunk in cupfuls 2 or 3 times daily

> Comfrey has gained prominence in the past quarter century for the remarkable results related from many places throughout the world in asthmatic complaints, gout, hay fever and the healing of old difficult sores.

ULCERS IN MOUTH AND LOOSE TEETH

PLANT: Acacia   *Acacia arabica*
WHERE FOUND: North Africa
PART USED: Bark
ACTION: Astringent
DISSERTATION: Joseph Miller writes, "It helps ulcers in the mouth and gums and fastens loose teeth."
METHOD: Bark has a high tannic acid content
DOSAGE: Use as a gargle in weak solution

ULCERS OF THE LOWER BOWELS AND COLITIS

PLANT: Monsonia   *Monsonia ovata*
WHERE FOUND: South Africa
PART USED: Whole plant
ACTION: Aromatic, astringent
DISSERTATION: It is highly recommended in South Africa for ulcerated conditions of the lower bowels. Good remedy also for acute and chronic dysentery.
METHOD: Tincture
DOSAGE: 1 ro 4 dr. every three to four hours

UNIVERSAL REMEDY

PLANT: Golden Seal   *Hydrastis canadensis*
WHERE FOUND: Eastern North America; now rarely found in native, but cultivated
PART USED: Rhizome, gathered in the fall of the year
ACTION: Alterative, detergent, laxative, tonic
DISSERTATION: Since about 1847 Golden Seal has figured

conspicuously in the botanic practice. The name was given to this plant by Thomsonians, who employed the root. The demand for "concentrations" was the means of discovering the two alkaloids contained in this drug — Hydrastine, the white, and Berberline, the yellow — besides others of less value. For many years these and the powdered root were the chief forms administered. Latterly, however, the drug in the form of a fluid extract is the most used and popular.

METHOD: Powdered Root — 1 tsp. to 1 pt. boiling water

DOSAGE: 1 to 2 tsp. 4 or 5 times a day

It is a very valuable remedy in disordered states of the digestive apparatus. As a general bitter tonic, it is applicable to debilitated conditions of mucous tissues. As a remedy for various gastric disorders it takes a leading place, acting very beneficially in acute inflammatory conditions. It will be found of value in all cases of dyspepsia, billiousness, and debility of the system. It is especially indicated in catarrhal states of the mucous membranes, gastric irritability, and passive hemmorrhages from the pelvic tissues. Externally it is used as a lotion in treatment of eye affections and as a general cleansing application.

URINARY, BLADDER AND KIDNEY COMPLAINTS

PLANT: Broom-Corn   *Sorghum vulgare*
WHERE FOUND: United States
PART USED: Seeds
ACTION: Demulcent, diuretic

DISSERTATION: The American negroes make a decoction and take it as a remedy for urinary, bladder and kidney disorders.
METHOD: 2 oz. of seeds with 1 qt. of water, boiled down to 1 pt.
DOSAGE: 1 tbs. in a glass of water at mealtimes

URINARY IRRITATION

PLANT: Arbutus, Trailing   *Epigaea repens*
WHERE FOUND: North America
PART USED: Herb (leaves)
ACTION: Astringent, diuretic
DISSERTATION: This plant is reputed to be superior to Uva-ursi in all afflictions of the urinary organs attended with irritation. It is also of value in gravel, debilitated or relaxed bladder, and in urine containing blood or pus.
METHOD: An infusion of 1 oz. of the leaves in 1 pt. boiling water
DOSAGE: Drink it freely

UTERINE TONIC, SEDATIVE, NERVINE

PLANT: Black Haw   *Viburnum prunifolium*
WHERE FOUND: Eastern and Central North America
PART USED: Bark of root
ACTION: Anti-spasmodic, nervine, sedative, uterine tonic
DISSERTATION: Much used for preventing miscarriage and should be given four or five weeks previous to the expected event. Checks pain and bleeding. An excellent remedy for dysmenorrhoea.
METHOD: An infusion of 1 oz. to 1 pt. boiling water
DOSAGE: Take in tablespoonful doses

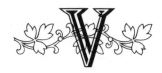

VALVULAR HEART DISEASE

PLANT: Lily of the Valley   *Convallaria majalis*
WHERE FOUND: Europe
PART USED: Flowers, leaves, whole plant
ACTION; Cardiac tonic, diuretic
DISSERTATION: Culpeper writes: "The herb is under the dominion of the moon and therefore cools and moistens like the former ... the syrup helps much to procure rest and to settle the brain of frantic persons, by cooling the hot temperature of the head. The distilled water of the flowers is very effectual ... and is recommended to take freckles, spots, sunburn and morphew from the face and other parts of the body.
METHOD: Infusion of ½ oz. of the herb to 1 pt. boiling water
DOSAGE: Tablespoonful doses

Large doses cause emesis and purgation. Has long been used in cardiac debility and dropsy. Its best use is for valvular heart disease.

VERMIN DESTROYER

PLANT: Sabadilla   *Schoenocaulon officinale*
WHERE FOUND: Guatemala, Mexico, Venezuela
PART USED: Seeds
ACTION: Acrid, bitter
DISSERTATION: It is used to destroy vermin
METHOD: Acetum (1 in 10)
        Ointment (1 in 4)

VERMIN DESTROYER

PLANT: Stavesacre   *Delphinium staphisagria*
WHERE FOUND: Greece, Italy, and Asia Minor
PART USED: Seeds
ACTION: Vermifuge
DISSERTATION: Thomas Green states in Universal Herbal:
"The common people use the powder of the seed to kill lice;
whence it is elegantly named lousewort. The seeds should be
sown where the plants are to remain. They are kept by druggists
and have been given in small doses against rheumatic and
venereal disorders; they vomit and purge, and that in so rough a
manner, that it is not safe to take them internally; when chewed
in the mouth, they excite a very large discharge of watery
humours from adjacent parts, and frequently prove serviceable
in disorders of the head, but are chiefly used to destroy the lice
with which children's heads are generally infested; and the
seeds, coarsely powdered and strewed among the hair, never
fails to remove them."

VERTIGO

PLANT: Woundwort   *Stachys palustris*
WHERE FOUND: Europe
PART USED: Herb
ACTION: Antiseptic, antispasmodic
DISSERTATION: An old remedy used to relieve cramp, pains in the joints, gout, falling sickness and vertigo. The bruised leaves when applied to a wound will arrest bleeding and heal the wound. The fresh juice is made into a syrup and taken internally to stop haemorrhages and dysentery.

Gerard writes of a case of a shoemaker's servant in Holborn "who intended to destroy himself. His attempt was thus: First he gave himself a most mortal wound in the throat in such sort that when I gave him drink it came forth at the wound which likewise did blow out the candle; another deep and grievous wound in the breast with the said dagger, and also two others 'in abdomine' or the nether belly ... which mortal wounds by God's permission and the virtues of this herb (woundwort) I perfectly cured within twenty days; for which the name of God be praised."

VITALITY, TO INCREASE

PLANT: Fo-Ti-Tieng or Gotu Kola   *Hydrocotyle asiatica*
WHERE FOUND: Asia and East Indies
PART USED: Leaves
ACTION: Aromatic, corrective, diuretic, nutritive, stimulant, tonic
DISSERTATION: Used in fevers, piles, bowel complaints and scrofulous conditions. Said to strengthen and energize the brain.
METHOD: A few leaves a day are taken, but just how they are

used I have been unable to discover. Presumably, they are chewed.

Many sensational claims have been made for this herb, among which are increased vitality, prolonging of life, effectiveness in leprosy, and great brain power. My studies have not justified these claims.

VOMITING

PLANT: Cascarilla   *Croton eleuteria*
WHERE FOUND: Jamaica and Bahamas
PART USED: Bark
ACTION: Aromatic, stimulant, tonic
DISSERTATION: Used in convalescence from acute diseases and to prevent vomiting. Also used in dyspepsia, flatulence and diarrhoea. When burnt, it gives off an aromatic odor and is thus used as a fumigant.
METHOD: Infusion of 1 oz. to 1 pt. boiling water
DOSAGE: Tablespoonful to a wineglassful as required

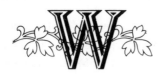

WARTS AND FUNGOID GROWTHS

PLANT: Thuja   *Thuja occidentalis*
WHERE FOUND: North America
PART USED: Leaves and tops
ACTION: Anthelmintic, emmenagogue, expectorant, irritant
DISSERTATION: Recommended in chronic coughs, fever, gout, amenorrhoea, etc. Externally it is used for removal of warts and fungoid growths.
METHOD: 1 oz. of herb in 1 pint of boiling water, taken internally
DOSAGE: Tablespoonful to wineglassful doses

WHITLOWS

PLANT: Whitlow-Grass or Nailwort   *Draba verna*
WHERE FOUND: Europe
PART USED: Herb
ACTION: Balsamic, diuretic
DISSERTATION: Culpeper states: "It is good for imposthumes in the joints and under the nails, called whitlows, felons, andicons, and nailwheals. It is an excellent wound herb, and under Jupiter. Inwardly taken, it is a balsamic medicine, a

remedy for the whites, and weaknesses occasioned by veneral disorders. It operates by urine, brings away gravel, and is good in disorders of the lungs."

WOMB DISEASE

PLANT: Dogwood or Red American Osier *Cornus sericea*
WHERE FOUND: North America
PART USED: Bark and bark of root
ACTION: Astringent, bitter, tonic
DISSERTATION: An infusion has been proven useful in checking vomiting due to pregnancy and disease of the womb. Has also been used in diarrhoea, dropsy, dyspepsia and fevers.
METHOD: Infusion of 1 oz. of bark in 1 pt. boiling water
DOSAGE: Tablespoonful 4 or 5 times a day, or more

WOUNDS

PLANT: Primrose *Primula vulgaris*
WHERE FOUND: English wild flowers
PART USED: Herb, root
ACTION: Antispasmodic, astringent, vermifuge

DISSERTATION: Culpeper states: "Of the leaves of Primroses is made as fine a salve to heal wounds as any that I know ... do not see your poor neighbours go with wounded limbs when an halfpenny cost will heal them."

In the early days of medicine, this plant constituted an important remedy in muscular rheumatism, paralysis and gout.

METHOD: Infusion of the root

DOSAGE: Tablespoonfuls

WRINKLES (Premature Aging)

PLANT: Oat groats   *Avena sativa*

WHERE FOUND: Temperate regions

PART USED: Seeds or groats

ACTION: Antispasmodic, corrective, nervine, nutritive, stimulant

DISSERTATION: Of much benefit in many conditions, febrile diseases, spermatorrhoea, insomnia, urinary problems, spasms, and strengthens heart muscles. An excellent restorative in exhaustion.

"Make a few small bags from cheesecloth; fill with oatmeal. Use instead of soap. Do not rinse the skin for two or three minutes after use; leave to dry, then rinse with water containing a few drops of tincture of Benzoin."

HERBAL COMPOUNDS

These herbal compounds from the archives of an old herbal family have been tested over the past 75 years. They claim these compounds have never failed; I am inclined to be less emphatic and say that they have seldom failed.

FOR GOUT AND RHEUMATISM

Couchgrass	½ oz.
Wood Betony	½ oz.
Prickly Ash Bark	½ oz.
Sarsaparilla Root	½ oz.
Guaiacum Raspings	¼ oz.

FOR BACKACHE AND THE KIDNEYS

Pellitory of the Wall	½ oz.
Parsley Piert or Buchu	½ oz.
Broom or Wild Carrot	½ oz.
Juniper Berries	½ oz.

BRONCHITIS COMPOUND

Hyssop	½ oz.
Comfrey Root	½ oz.
Horehound	½ oz.
Coltsfoot Leaves	½ oz.
Liquorice Juice	¼ oz.

COLDS AND INFLUENZA COMPOUND

Yarrow	½ oz.
Peppermint	½ oz.
Elder Flowers	½ oz.
Chillies	½ doz.

FOR VARIOUS NERVE TROUBLES

Scullcap	½ oz.
Mistletoe	½ oz.
Wood Betony (or Vervain)	½ oz.
Peruvian Bark	¼ oz.

BLOOD PURIFYING COMPOUND

Sarsaparilla Root	½ oz.
Burdock Root	½ oz.
Sassafras Bark	½ oz.
Yellow Dock Root	½ oz.

STOMACH AND LIVER COMPOUND

Barberry Bark	½ oz.
Agrimony	½ oz.
Centaury	½ oz.
Meadowsweet	½ oz.
Ginger Root, crushed	¼ oz.

To any of the afore mentioned compounds, add two pints of cold water, bring to the boil and gently simmer (with lid on) for 10 minutes. Allow to cool. The Cold and Influenza Compound should be taken freely if the patient remains indoors.

SORE THROAT AND GARGLE COMPOUND

For all sore throats, quinsies, etc. Far safer and far better than all the antibiotics, with NO side effects.

Ragwort	½ oz.
Red Sage	½ oz.
Chillies	½ doz.

Pour over one pint of boiling water. When cold, pour off approximately half the liquid into another jug and add to this four tablespoonsful (2 oz.) Cider Vinegar. This should be used as a gargle freely. The other half still standing on the herbs should be taken as a medicine, two tablespoonfuls three times daily.

AROMATIC

Sage	½ oz.
Rosemary	½ oz.
Thyme	½ oz.
Wild Thyme	½ oz.
Hyssop	½ oz.
Marjoram	½ oz.
Wormwood	½ oz.
Peppermint	½ oz.

Prepare as an infusion.

FOR HEADACHE

Rosemary	½ oz.
Thyme	½ oz.
Wild Thyme	½ oz.
Wild Marjoram	½ oz.
Peppermint	½ oz.
Lavender Flowers	½ oz.
Rose Flowers	½ oz.
Marjoram	½ oz.

Prepare as an infusion.

COUGH

Maidenhair	½ oz.
Hart's Tongue	½ oz.
Poppy Capsules	½ oz.
Vervain	½ oz.
Hyssop	½ oz.
Ground Ivy	½ oz.

Prepare as an infusion.

TONIC FOR INFANTS

Fennel	½ oz.
Aniseed	½ oz.
Couchgrass	1 oz.
Polypody	1 oz.
Liquorice Root	2 oz.
Figs	2 oz.
John's Bread	2 oz.
Lime Flowers	2 oz.
Hartshorn	2 oz.

Prepare as an infusion.

FOR CHEST AND LUNGS

Marshmallow Flowers	½ oz.
Mallow Flowers	½ oz.
Coltsfoot Flowers	½ oz.
Violet Flowers	½ oz.
Mullein Flowers	½ oz.
Red Poppy Flowers	½ oz.
Catsfoot Flowers	½ oz.

Prepare as an infusion.

TO EXPEL WORMS

Tansy	½ oz.
Wormwood	½ oz.
Wormseed (Levant)	½ oz.
Chamomile	½ oz.

Prepare as an infusion.

HEALTH TEA

Fennel	½ oz.
Cream of Tartar	½ oz.
Elder Flowers	1 oz.
Aniseed	1 oz.
Senna Leaves	2 oz.

Prepare as an infusion.

A SOOTHING COMPOUND

Marshmallow Flowers	½ oz.
Mallow Flowers	½ oz.
Mullein Flowers	½ oz.
Pellitory-of-the-Wall	½ oz.

Prepare as an infusion.

TO ASSIST MENSTRUATION

Black Hellebore Root	½ oz.
Valerian Root	½ oz.
Mugwort Herb	½ oz.
Wormwood Herb	½ oz.
Wormseed	½ oz.

Prepare as a decoction.

TO INCREASE THE FLOW OF URINE

Asparagus Root	½ oz.
Parsley Root	½ oz.
Celery Root	½ oz.
Fennel	½ oz.
Butcher's Broom	½ oz.

Prepare as a decoction.

TO CAUSE SWEATING

Marshmallow Root	4 oz.
Liquorice Root	2 oz.
Orris Root	2 oz.
Ground Ivy	2 oz.
Aniseed	½ oz.
Coltsfoot Leaves	2 oz.
Red Poppy Flowers	1 oz.
Mullein	1 oz.

Prepare as an infusion.

TO RESTORE NORMAL FUNCTIONS OF THE BODY

Sassafras Wood	½ oz.
Elder Flowers	½ oz.
Red Poppy Flowers	½ oz.
Borage Leaves	½ oz.

Prepare as an infusion.

TO EXPEL WIND AND EASE GRIPING PAINS

Aniseed	½ oz.
Fennel	½ oz.
Caraway	½ oz.
Coriander	½ oz.

Prepare as an infusion.

TO STIMULATE THE APPETITE

Holy Thistle	½ oz.
Germander	½ oz.
Centaury	½ oz.
Buckbean	½ oz.

Prepare as an infusion.

TO PREVENT OR STOP SPASM

Yarrow Herb	½ oz.
Orange Flowers	1 oz.
Valerian Root	1½ oz.

Prepare as an infusion.

TO COUNTERACT CATARRH

Goosefoot   ½ oz.
Rupturewort   ½ oz.

Prepare as an infusion.
FOR CONSTIPATION

Wormwood   ½ oz.
Wood Betony   ½ oz.
Bugle   ½ oz.
Mountain Mint   ½ oz.
Water Germander   ½ oz.
Hyssop   ½ oz.
Ground Ivy   ½ oz.
Yarrow   ½ oz.
Marjoram   ½ oz.
Periwinkle   ½ oz.
Rosemary   ½ oz.
Sanicle   ½ oz.
Sage   ½ oz.
Thyme   ½ oz.
Wild Thyme   ½ oz.
Germander   ½ oz.
Vervain   ½ oz.
Arnica Flowers   ½ oz.
Catsfoot Flowers   ½ oz.
Coltsfoot Flowers   ½ oz.

Prepare as an infusion.
FOR SEXUAL DEBILITY

Kola   1 oz.
Damiana   1 oz.
Saw Palmetto   1 oz.

Use fluid extract, 1 oz. of each, mixed together. Dosage: Small teaspoonful three times a day.

FOR HAEMORRHOIDS OR PILES

Pilewort	1 oz.
Yarrow	1 oz.
Senna Pods	1 oz.
Guaiacum Chips	2 oz.
Poplar Bark	1 oz.
Raisins	2 oz.

Boil in 4 pints of water and simmer down to 1 pint. Take a tablespoonful three times a day.

FOR BLEEDING PILES

Silver Weed	2 oz.
Tormentil Root	1 oz.

Boil in 2 pints of water and take a tablespoonful three times a day.

FOR HIVES

Stinging Nettles	1 oz.
Yarrow	1 oz.
Golden Seal	¼ oz.
Dandelion Root	2 oz.

Simmer for 20 minutes in 2 pints of water and take a tablespoonful every four hours.

OVARIAN CYSTS

Liquorice Root	2 oz.
Yarrow	1 oz.
Comfrey	1 oz.
Yellow Dock	1 oz.
Dandelion	1 oz.

Boil in a pint of water for an hour, strain and take one tablespoonful three times daily.

NEURASTHENIA

Lady's Slipper	1 oz.
Vervain	1 oz.
Valerian	1 oz.
Scullcap	1 oz.
Saw Palmetto	1 oz.
Raspberry Leaves	1 oz.
Peruvian Bark	1 oz.
Liverwort	1 oz.
Kola Nuts	1 oz.
Barberry Bark	1 oz.
Mistletoe	1 oz.

Add 5 pints of water and simmer down to 2 pints, and add ½ oz. of Essence of Cayenne. Take one tablespoonful three times a day after meals.

HEPATITIS

Yarrow	1 oz.
Liverwort	1 oz.
Barberry	1 oz.
Centuary	1 oz.
Dandelion	1 oz.
Lobelia	1 oz.

Boil in 3 pints of water and simmer down to 1 pint, and add 1 oz. of Tincture of Rhubarb. Dose: One tablespoonful every four hours.

FOR TOXIC CONDITION OF THE BODY

Yellow Dock	½ oz.
Queen's Delight	½ oz.

Make an infusion, using one pint of boiling water, and take wineglassful doses several times daily after food.

FOR SYNOVITIS

Poppy Heads	½ oz.
Chamomile	½ oz.

In this painful condition fomentations of Poppy heads and Chamomile flowers are most helpful. Apply several times daily. Alternate hot and cold compresses should be used as part of the treatment.

FOR REMOVING PROUD FLESH

Raspberry Leaves	½ oz.
Slippery Elm, powdered bark	½ oz.

Make into a poultice and apply to the affected parts.

FOR HELP IN MENOPAUSE

Clivers	1 oz.
Wood Betony	1 oz.
Sanicle	1 oz.
Chamomile	1 oz.

Prepare as an infusion - 1 oz. to 1 pt. of water. Take wineglassful doses after meals. Keep the bowels open.

FOR MIGRAINE

Golden Seal	1 oz.
Dandelion Root	1 oz.
American Mandrake	½ oz.

Decoction. Take in wineglassful doses half an hour before food.

FOR ERYSIPELAS

Clivers	1 oz.
Elder leaves	1 oz.

Mix and prepare an infusion with 1½ pts. of boiling water. Take frequent wineglassful doses.

HERBS USED IN CANCER

These herbs and foods, I have found, have been used in the treatment of cancer throughout the world. Many of them have brought varying results. Practitioners of many fields of healing have claimed cures by their use; and I am unable to prove or disprove these claims.

Because of the controversial nature of various cancer treatments and cancer cures I hesitated publishing this list. However, after careful consideration of all aspects, I decided that where so many lives are at stake it is my duty to make public any form of natural treatment that might be of help. Therefore I present this list without prejudice.

PLANT: Alehoof or Ground Ivy   *Glechoma hederacea*
WHERE FOUND: Europe
PART USED: Herb
PLANT: Red or Purple Clover   *Trifolium pratense*
WHERE FOUND: Worldwide
PART USED: Flower
PLANT: Cocklebur or Stickwort   *Agrimonia eupatoria*
WHERE FOUND: Europe
PART USED: Herb

PLANT: Deadly Nightshade or Dwale   *Atropa belladonna*
WHERE FOUND: Europe and Asia
PART USED: Root and leaves
PLANT: Poison Hemlock   *Conium maculatum*
WHERE FOUND: Europe
PART USED: Leaves and unripe fruit
PLANT: Clivers or Goosegrass   *Galium aparine*
WHERE FOUND: Europe
PART USED: Herb
PLANT: Buckbean or Marsh Trefoil   *Menyanthes trifoliata*
WHERE FOUND: Europe, Asia and North America
PART USED: Herb
PLANT: Field Elm   *Ulmus campestris*
WHERE FOUND: Britain
PART USED: Bark
PLANT: May Apple or Mandrake   *Podophyllum peltatum*
WHERE FOUND: North America
PART USED: Rhizome
PLANT: Scotch Thistle   *Onopordum acanthium*
WHERE FOUND: Europe
PART USED: Herb
PLANT: Biting Stonecrop or Wall Pepper   *Sedum acre*
WHERE FOUND: Europe, Asia and North America
PART USED: Herb
PLANT: Violet   *Viola odorata*
WHERE FOUND: Europe, Asia and Africa
PART USED: Leaves
PLANT: Blessed Thistle   *Cnicus benedictus*
WHERE FOUND: Mediterranean, Caucasus and N. America
PART USED: Herb
PLANT: Greater Celandine   *Chelidonium majus*
WHERE FOUND: Europe
PART USED: Herb
PLANT: Sweet Marjoram   *Origanum majorana*
WHERE FOUND: Mediterranean and Europe
PART USED: Leaves and herb

PLANT: Comfrey   *Symphytum officinale*
WHERE FOUND: Europe, Asia and North America
PART USED: Leaves and root
PLANT: Golden Seal   *Hydrastis canadensis*
WHERE FOUND: North America
PART USED: Rhizome
PLANT: Rue or Ave-Grace   *Ruta graveolens*
WHERE FOUND: Europe and North America
PART USED: Herb
PLANT: Burdock   *Arctium lappa*
WHERE FOUND: Europe and North America
PART USED: Herb, root, seeds (fruit)
PLANT: Yellow Dock   *Rumex crispus*
WHERE FOUND: Europe and North America
PART USED: Root
PLANT: Dandelion   *Taraxacum officinale*
WHERE FOUND: Worldwide
PART USED: Root
PLANT: Blue Flag   *Iris versicolor*
WHERE FOUND: North America
PART USED: Rhizome
PLANT: Wood Betony   *Stachys betonica*
WHERE FOUND: Europe and Asia
PART USED: Herb
PLANT: Rock Rose   *Helianthemum canadense*
WHERE FOUND: North America
PART USED: Herb
PLANT: Periwinkle or Vinca Rosea   *Vinca minor*
WHERE FOUND: Europe, cultivated worldwide
PART USED: Herb
PLANT: Parsley   *Carum petroselinum*
WHERE FOUND: Worldwide
PART USED: Leaves, root, seeds
PLANT: Grape   *Vitis vinifera and labrasca*
WHERE FOUND: Europe and North America

PART USED: Fruit
COMMODITY: Powdered Egg Shells

Regarding grapes, I might mention that a book which has been published in at least 24 editions from 1928 to 1968, called "The Grape Cure" and written by Johanna Brandt, tells the story of how she cured herself of cancer and then helped innumerable others heal themselves by a strict diet of grapes. I can attest to the fact that thousands have taken this treatment. At least three medical doctors have given testimony in writing to the value of her treatment.

In one chapter she says: "Germany seems to be the centre of this natural healing cult. The grape diet is recommended by Dr. Herman Reider, University Professor, and Dr. Martin Zeller, both of Munchen, Germany. For a complete cure these doctors prescribe the juice of freshly pressed grapes to be taken in five meals daily. Their treatment lasts from four to six weeks and the best time to undergo it is during September and October. In some cases large quantities of juice are administered ... from two pounds to thirteen pounds of pressed grapes being used daily. (We do not recommend the consumption of more than four pounds of grapes daily under most circumstances.)"

In his Family Botanic Guide, published in 1907, under the heading of Cancer, Wm. Fox, M.D. states:

"Cancers are ulcers of the very worst kind, and proceed from a poison or virus in the blood, forming morbid matter which is sent among the glands and other vascular portions of the system. This accumulates by degrees, though it remains nearly unchanged, till by its obstruction to the circulation and the nervous action in the part, it gives power to the inorganic agencies to produce lesions, which are fatal when the system cannot remove the offensive matter. Various applications are

192

recommended and used for cancers by medical men; but the knife is employed as the principal remedy, yet I have never seen a solitary instance cured by it. Dr. Munro states 'that out of nearly sixty cases of extirpation of cancer at which he was present, only four patients remained free of the disease at the end of two years.' Dr. Jackson, of Boston, America, in his lectures on Morbid Anatomy, stated that after a cancer has been operated upon with the knife it returns in a short time with great malignity, and attacks other organs and parts of the body.

"SYMPTOMS — The breast is often the seat of this complaint, but other parts are liable to become affected. When the female breast is affected, there is a moveable hard tumour about the size of a marble. When in this stage it progresses slowly, attended with an uneasiness in the part affected, but without inflammation; it gradually increases in size, and becomes hard and knotty to the touch. As it progresses further there is a darting and burning pain felt in the tumour, and it becomes attached to the skin above and to the parts beneath, converting the whole into one common mass. Before it has attained any great size, there is a discharge of dark-coloured and offensive matter. The discharge is so acrid as to inflame the parts it comes in contact with. The ulcer now spreads rapidly, and unless it be checked it corrupts the whole stream of life, and the patient is so reduced that it frequently terminates fatally.

"TREATMENT — Means must be adopted to improve the general health of the sufferer. Give the following decoction:

Quassia chips	1 oz.
Yellow dock root	1 oz.
Bittersweet(American)	1 oz.
Cinquefoil	1 oz.
Agrimony	1 oz.

Add two quarts of water, and boil down to three pints, then add a teaspoonful of cayenne, and, when cold, two ounces of the decoction of red Jamaica sarsaparilla. Take a wineglassful three times a day. Then poultice the cancer with the green herb called spotted hemlock, bruised with a hammer very fine, spread on a cloth, and apply to the part affected several times a day; if a bleeding cancer, use freely of powdered Peruvian bark and gum myrrh before applying the poultice. Care must be taken with the hemlock, as it is poisonous. When the cancer is foetid and emits an offensive smell, a charcoal poultice can be applied with great advantage. Simmer half a pint of yeast in the oven, and while it remains hot mix the charcoal with the yeast until it is of a proper consistency. Poultice the cancer as often as required; place a thin gauze or muslin upon the cancer before applying the poultice. This process will stimulate the absorbents to take up the foreign deposit; but if the tumour has advance too far, poultice it with slippery elm, lobelia and blood root in equal parts, at the same time washing the breast with bark tea. If this be persevered with, it will never, or seldom, fail to cure. The following is a very good cancer liniment of great power:

Tincture of blue flag	2 oz.
Tincture of blood root	1 oz.
Tincture of red clover	1 oz.

Mix them all together, then saturate a cloth in the solution and apply it twice a day. We have seldom known this to fail. Sometimes use the spotted hemlock and at others use the poultice. They will all work together well. Cancers in the early stages have been cured by simply washing the ulcer with a strong decoction of the root of the yellow dock, applied as warm as the patient could bear it. Wash and scrape the roots of fresh docks fine, and lay on the cancer as a poultice; keep them moist, and change them five or six times a day."

Here are two additional remedies taken from another old herbal:

FOR BREAST CANCER

Phytolacca	2 oz.
Gentian	1 oz.
Dandelion Root	1 oz.

Boil in three pints of water and simmer to one pint. Make a simple syrup with honey. One teaspoonful after each meal is recommended.

FOR SKIN CANCER (OINTMENT)

Make a very strong tea with red clover blossoms and violet leaves and flowers. The tea is then strained and the liquid is simmered slowly until it is of the consistency of tar. This same ointment was used to remove tumours.

GUIDE TO THERAPEUTIC ACTION

ALTERATIVE: Blue Flag, Burdock, Echinacea, Figwort, Mezereon, Poke Root, Queen's Delight, Red Clover, Sarsaparilla, Turkey Corn, Yellow Duck.

ANODYNE: Aconite, Coca, Henbane, Hops, Indian Hemp, Jamaica Dogwood, Poppy.

ANTHELMINTIC: Aloes, Butternut, Kousso, Male Fern, Pinkroot, Tansy, Wormseed, Wormwood.

ANTIBILIOUS: Balmony, American Mandrake, Wild Yam.

ANTIPERIODIC: Alstonia, Ash, Cinchona, Feverbush, Quebracho, Wafer Ash, White Willow.

ANTISCORBUTIC: Lemon, Lime Fruit, Scurvy-Grass, Shepherd's Purse.

ANTISCROFULOUS: American Adder's Tongue.

ANTISEPTIC: Barberry, Echinacea, Eucalyptus, Golden Seal, Southernwood, Thyme, White Pond Lily, Wild Indigo.

ANTISPASMODIC: Asafoetida, Black Haw, Chamomile, Black Cohosh, Cramp Bark, Gelsemium, Lady's Slipper, Lobelia, Mistletoe, Pulsatilla, Skullcap, Stramonium, Sundew, Valerian.

APERIENT: Rhubarb, Pale Rose.

APHRODISIAC: Damiana, Muirapuama, Saw Palmetto, Yohimbe Bark.

AROMATIC: Allspice, European Angelica, Angostura, Basil, Bugle, Burnet Saxifrage, Calamus, Canella, Cinnamon, Condurango, Cubeb, Golden Rod, Magnolia, Meadowsweet, Melilot, Musk Seed, Orange, Summer Savory, Tonka Beans, Winter's Bark.

ASTRINGENT: Avens, Bayberry, Bistort, Blackberry, Catechu, Cranesbill, Nettle, Oak, Pinus Bark, Rhatany, Tormentilla, Witch Hazel.

BALSAMIC: Clary, Larch.

BITTER: Angostura, Bugle, Canchalagua, Cascara Amarga, Cedron, Chiretta, Feverfew, Gentian, Gold Thread, Horehound, American Red Osier, Quassia.

CARDIAC: Asparagus, European Birch, Butterbur, Foxglove, Hawthorn, American Hellebore, False Hellebore, Kola, Lily-of-the-Valley, Mescal Buttons, Mountain Laurel, Night-Blooming Cereus, Strophanthus, Tonka Beans, Tree of Heaven.

CARMINATIVE: Allspice, Angelica, Aniseed, Balm, Calamus, Cinnamon, Cloves, Fennel, Ginger, Peppermint.

CATHARTIC: American Black Alder, Bitter Apple, Black Root, Broom, White Bryony, Alder, Buckthorn, Butternut, Cabbage Tree, Castor Oil, Colchicum, Copaiba, Croton, Dyer's Greenweed, Gladwin, Hedge-Hyssop, Black Hellebore, Hemp, Agrimony, Holly, Hydrangea, Indian Physic, Ivy, Jalap, American Mandrake, Mountain Flax, Poke Root, Rhubarb, Senna, Squill, Swamp Milkweed, Turpeth.

CORRECTIVE: Oliver Bark.

DEMULCENT: Arrowroot, Comfrey, Couchgrass, Iceland Moss, Irish Moss, Linseed, Liquorice Root, Marshmallow, Slippery Elm.

DEOBSTRUENT: Bladderwrack, Buckbean, Butcher's Broom, Eternal Flower, English Liverwort, Water Dock, Wild Carrot.

DEPURATIVE: Figwort.

DERMATIC: Chaulmoogra.

DETERGENT: English Adder's Tongue, Balmony, Black Currant, Goa, Golden Seal, Ragwort, Soap Tree, Soapwort, Southernwood, Walnut, Water Betony, Water Dock.

DIAPHORETIC AND SUDORIFIC: Angelica, Balm, Boneset, Crawley Root, Ipecacuanha, Jaborandi, Pennyroyal, Prickly Ash, Yarrow.

DIGESTIVE: Paw-Paw, Paw-Paw Seed.

DIURETIC: Broom, Buchu, Clivers, Couchgrass, Hydrangea, Juniper Berries, Pareira, Parsley, Parsley Piert, Pellitory, Pipsissiwa, Shepherd's Purse, Stone Root, Uva-Ursi, Wild Carrot.

EMETIC: Bitter Root, Ipecacuanha, Lobelia, Mustard, Tag Alder, Vervain.

EMMENAGOGUE: Aloes, Arrach, Black Cohosh, Blue Cohosh, Corn Ergot, Ergot, Ground Pine, Black Hellebore, Life Root, Motherwort, Mugwort, Pennyroyal, Rue, Southernwood, Tansy, Wood Sage.

EMOLLIENT: Linseed, Liquorice Root, Marshmallow, Slippery Elm.

EXPECTORANT: Benzoin, Elecampane, Horehound, Ipecacuanha, Lobelia, Lungwort, Mouse-Ear, Mullein, Pleurisy Root, Polypody Root, Senega, Squill, Wild Cherry, Yerba Santa.

FEBRIFUGE AND REFRIGERANT: Aconite, Angostura, Alstonia, Avens, Balm, Boneset, Catnip, Crawley Root, Devil's Bit, Five-leaf Grass, Gelsemium, American Hellebore, Peruvian Bark, Wormwood.

HEMOSTATIC: Bistort, Cranesbill, Corn Ergot, Ergot.

HEPATIC: Dodder, Pichi, Yellow Toadflax.

HYDROGOGUE: White Bryony, American Mandrake.

HYPNOTIC AND NARCOTIC: Belladonna, Bittersweet, Bugleweed, Hemlock, Henbane, Indian Hemp, Mistletoe, Passion Flower, Poppy, Stramonium.

INSECTICIDE: Musk Seed, Pyrethrum.

IRRITANT: Bitter Apple Bryony, Cayenne, Mustard, Poison Oak, Thuja.

LAXATIVE: Buckthorn, Cascara Sagrada, Dandelion, Golden Seal, Mandrake, Manna, Mountain Flax.

MYDRIATIC: Belladonna, Henbane, Stramonium.

MYOTIC: Calabar Bean.

NERVINE: Arrach, Black Haw, Cramp Bark, Guarana, Kola, Lady's Slipper, Lime Flowers, Mistletoe, Motherwort, Muira-Puama, Oats, Pulsatilla, Skullcap, Snake Root, Sumbul, Valerian, Vervain.

NUTRITIVE: Arrowroot, Iceland Moss, Irish Moss, Salep, Saw Palmetto, Slippery Elm.

OXYTOCIC: Cotton Root.

PARASITICIDE: Cocculus indicus.

PARTURIENT: Corn Ergot, Cotton Root, Squaw Vine.

PECTORAL: Aniseed, Beth Root, Blue Mallow, Euphorbia, Hartstongue, Hyssop, Irish Moss, Jujube Berries, Labrador Tea, Life Root, Linseed, Liquorice Root, American Liverwort, Lungwort, Maiden Hair, Mullein, Polypody Root, American Sarsaparilla, Slippery Elm, Sundew, Wild Cherry.

PURGATIVE: Aloes, Bitter Apple, Jalap, Mandrake, Scammony.

RESOLVENT: Bittersweet, Galbanum.

RUBEFACIENT: Black Bryony, Cayenne, Cowhage, Croton, Pellitory, Pine Oil, Turpentine.

STERNUTATORY: Asarabacca, Egyptian Soapwort Root.

STIMULANT: Ammoniac, Blood Root, Cascarilla, Cayenne, Cinnamon, Cloves, Ginger, Horseradish, Jaborandi, Kola, Mustard, Nux Vomica, Paraguay Tea, Pennyroyal, Peppermint, Peruvian Balsam, Poplar, Prickly Ash, Snake Root, Wintergreen.

STOMACHIC: Allspice, Avens, Calamus, Centaury, Chamomile, Condurango, Cubebs, Peppermint, Quassia, Rhubarb, True Unicorn Root.

STYPTIC: Avens, American Cranebill Root, Lady's Mantle.

SUDORIFIC: American Sarsaparilla, Vervain.

TAENIFUGE: Kamala, Kousso, Male Fern.

TONIC: Alstonia, Barberry, Bitter Root, Buckbean, Calumba, Chamomile, Chiretta, Centaury, Damiana, Gentian, Gold Thread, Hops, Kola, Nux Vomica, Peruvian Bark, Pipsissiwa, Poplar, Prickly Ash, Quassia, Strophanthus, Turkey Corn, Unicorn Root, Wild Cherry, Wormwood.

VERMIFUGE: Butternut, Cabbage Tree, Blue Cohosh, Corsican Moss, Goat's Rue, Black Horehound, Male Fern, Pink Root, Primrose, Stavesacre, Wormseed.

VULNERARY: Arnica, Crosswort, Myrrh, Water Betony

FORMS OF BOTANICAL
MEDICINAL PREPARATIONS

INFUSIONS

These preparations are generally made of ground or bruised roots, barks, herbs, or seeds, by pouring boiling water over the drug, letting it stand for half an hour, occasionally stirring, and finally straining the clear liquid carefully off. Sometimes cold water may be used, as in the case of a few bitters, such as Calumba, Quassia, etc., when the ground drug will be found to yield its properties to water without heat. The usual quantity of drug to 1 pint of water is 1 oz., but in a few cases where the drugs contain very active principles, less is sufficient. The dose of most infusions varies from a tablespoonful to a wineglassful or a teacupful.

DECOCTIONS

As a rule decoctions are made by pouring cold water upon the cut, bruised, or ground drug, the mixture being boiled for twenty minutes to half an hour, cooled and strained. Roots and barks are generally treated in this manner, as they need longer subjection to heat to extract their virtues. Decoctions are generally made in a strength of 1 oz. to 1 pt., but, as the water boils away, it is best to use 1½ pt., and the decoctions should then, when finished, measure 1 pt. The length of time depends upon the readiness with which the drug gives up its active principles to the liquid. The dose varies from two teaspoonfuls to a wineglassful or two.

LIQUID EXTRACTS

These are most popular and convenient preparations inasmuch as, if properly made, they are the most concentrated fluid forms in which vegetable drugs may be obtained. Liquid extracts are made in a variety of ways — evaporation by heat, in vacuo; cold percolation; high pressure, etc. — each drug being treated in that manner by which its properties may best be extracted and held in concentrated solution. The strength of a Liquid extract is 1 in 1, or 1 oz. fluid represents 1 oz. of crude drug — for instance, 1 oz. of Liquid Ext. Golden Seal would represent the medicinal value of 1 oz. of Golden Seal Root. Liquid extracts are daily becoming more popular, and, as they may be easily obtained, bid fair to rival the Tinctures and Preparations which have made Homoeopathy so popular with those who seek an easy way of keeping a household stock of domestic remedies.

SOLID EXTRACTS

Are prepared by evaporating to the consistence of honey the fresh juices or strong infusions of vegetable drugs. They may also be manufactured by spirituous process, in which case the alcohol is recovered by means of distillation from a strong tincture of the drug. Solid extracts are employed chiefly in the manufacture of pills, plasters, ointments, and compressed tablets.

TINCTURES

Are spirituous preparations made with pure or diluted spirits of wine of drugs containing gummy, resinous, or volatile principles, or of any drugs rendered useless by the application of heat in any form, or of the great number of drugs which will not yield their properties to water alone, as their active principles are more readily extracted by spirit, better held in solution and preserved from deterioration.

Tinctures are generally made in a strength of 1 or 2 oz. of drug to 1 pt. The dose varies according to the active principles contained in the drug.

PILLS

Are perhaps the best known and most largely used form of medicines, chiefly because of their handy form and general convenience, and also because of their comparative tastelessness. Pills are for the most part composed of concentrated extracts and alkaloids in combination with active crude drugs. They may be obtained coated or uncoated, but the pearl-coated pill is the general favourite, as it is quite tasteless, and the coating, if properly made, is readily soluble in the stomach.

TABLETS

Are made by compressing drugs into a very small compass. It is claimed for them that they are superior to pills, because they are more easily administered and by reason of their rapid dissolution in the stomach are quicker in their action.

CAPSULES

Are gelatine containers of convenient sizes for swallowing and holding oils, balsams, etc., which, because of their nauseous taste or smell, would be difficult to administer. Such drugs as Cod Liver Oil, Castor Oil, Copaiba, Sandalwood Oil, etc., are largely given in this form, because objection is made to the remedies in their natural state.

SUPPOSITORIES

Are small cones made of some convenient and easily soluble base, and used where it is desired to apply medicines per rectum. They are invaluable in the treatment of internal piles, cancers, fistula, etc. They are also made of nutrient ingredients, and passed into the bowels where patients are unable to take nourishment in the usual manner.

PESSARIES

Are similar to Suppositories, but are made in a suitable shape to be used in female complaints, where it is desirable to apply remedies to the walls of the internal passages.

CONCENTRATIONS

Are a class of medicinal resins or resinoids obtained from medicinal drugs by precipitation from their alcoholic preparations, either by water, distillation, or other suitable means.

Those at present in use contain one or more, but not always all the therapeutic virtues of the drugs from which they are made, and in many cases are only powdered extracts.

DEFINITIONS OF HERBAL
MEDICAL TERMS

ALEXIPHARMIC: Capable of warding off or resisting poisons.

ALTERATIVE: A medicine that alters the processes of nutrition and excretion, restoring the normal functions of the system.

ANODYNE: An agent that will relieve pain; milder in form than an analgesic.

ANTHELMINTIC: An agent used to expel intestinal worms.

ANTIBILIOUS: Relieving bilious conditions.

ANTIPHLOGISTIC: Capable of relieving inflammation.

ANTIPERIODIC: Antimalarial; preventing regular recurrences.

ANTISCORBUTIC: An agent effective against or a remedy for scurvy.

ANTISCROFULOUS: An agent effective against or a remedy for scrofula.

ANTISEPTIC: (a) Preventing decay, putrefaction, or sepsis. (b) An agent that will prevent the growth or arrest the development of microorganisms.

ANTISPASMODIC: (a) Relieving or checking spasm. (b) An agent that will relieve spasm.

APERIENT: A very mild laxative.

APHRODISIAC: An agent which stimulates sexual desire.

AROMATIC: (a) Having an agreeable odor. (b) Belonging to that series of carbon compounds in which the carbon atoms form closed rings (as in benzene) as distinguished from the aliphatic series in which the atoms form straight or branched chains.

ASTRINGENT: (a) Drawing together, constricting, binding. (b) An agent that has a constricting or binding effect, e.g., one which checks hemorrhages, secretion, etc.

BALSAMIC: (a) Pertaining to balsam. (b) Aromatic.

BITTER: Having a disagreeable taste.

CARDIAC: (a) Pertaining to the heart or to the cardiac orifice into the stomach. (b) Having heart disease. (c) A heart tonic.

CARMINATIVE: An agent that will remove gases from the gastrointestinal tract.

CATHARTIC: An active purgative, usually producing several evacuations which may or may not be accompanied by pain or tenesmus.

CORRECTIVE: (a) A drug that modifies action of another. (b) Pertaining to such a drug.

DEMULCENT: An agent that will soothe the part or soften the skin to which applied. The term is usually restricted to agents acting on mucous membrane.

DEOBSTRUENT: Having the property of removing obstructions.

DEPURATIVE: Cleansing.

DERMATIC: An agent effective against dermatitis or other skin conditions.

DETERGENT: (a) A medicine that purges or cleanses; cleansing. (b) A cleaning agent prepared synthetically from higher alcohols, sulfuric acid and caustic soda.

DIAPHORETIC: A sudorific or an agent which increases perspiration. The term sudorific is usually confined to those active agents that cause drops of perspiration to collect on the skin.

DIGESTIVE: An agent effective against digestive disorders; an aid to digestion.

DIURETIC: Increasing or an agent which increases the secretion of urine.

EMETIC: Medicine that induces vomiting.

EMMENAGOGUE: An agent that stimulates the menstrual function.

EMOLLIENT: An agent that will soften and soothe the part when applied locally. The term is usually confined to agents affecting the surface of the body.

EXPECTORANT: An agent that facilitates the removal of the secretions of the bronchopulmonary mucous membrane. Expectorants are sometimes classed as sedative expectorants and stimulating expectorants.

FEBRIFUGE: That which lessens fever.

HEMOSTATIC: (a) Checking hemmorrhage. (b) Any substance which checks bleeding without being directly applied to the bleeding areas.

HEPATIC: Pertaining to the liver.

HYDROGOGUE: An agent for conveying water.

HYPNOTIC: (a) Pertaining to sleep or hypnosis. (b) An agent that induces sleep or which dulls the senses.

INSECTICIDE: (a) An agent used to exterminate insects. (b) Destructive to insects.

IRRITANT: An agent which, when used locally, produces more or less local inflammatory reaction. Anything which induces or gives rise to irritation.

LAXATIVE: A mildly purgative medicine; an aperient or mild cathartic producing one or two evacuations without pain or tenesmus.

MYDRIATIC: (a) Causing pupillary dilatation. (b) Any drug which dilates the pupil.

MYOTIC: (a) An agent that will contract the pupil of the eye. (b) Producing contraction of a pupil.

NARCOTIC: (a) Producing stupor or sleep. (b) A drug which in moderate doses depresses the central nervous system thus relieving pain and producing sleep but which in excessive dose produces unconsciousness, stupor, coma, and possibly death. (c) Anything that soothes, relieves or lulls. (d) One addicted to the use of narcotics.

NERVINE: (a) Acting as a nerve sedative. (b) An agent that lessens irritability of nerves and increases nerve energy.

NUTRITIVE: Pertaining to the process of assimilating food; having the property of nourishing.

OXYTOCIC: (a) An agent which stimulates uterine contractions. (b) Accelerating childbirth.

PARASITICIDE: (a) Killing parasites. (b) An agent that will kill parasites.

PARTURIENT: (a) Concerning childbirth or parturition. (b) Bringing forth; giving birth.

PECTORAL: (a) Concerning the chest. (b) Efficacious in relieving chest conditions, as a cough.

PURGATIVE: (a) Cleansing. (b) An agent that will cause watery evacuation of the intestinal contents.

REFRIGERANT: (a) Allaying heat or fever; cooling. (b) Medicine or agent which relieves thirst and is cooling or reduces a fever.

RESOLVENT: (a) Promoting disappearance of inflammation. (b) That which causes dispersion of inflammation.

RUBEFACIENT: (a) Causing redness, as of the skin. (b) Agent which reddens the skin, producing a local congestion, the vessels becoming dilated and the supply of blood increased.

STERNUTATORY: Causing sneezing.

STIMULANT: Any agent temporarily increasing functional activity.

STOMACHIC: (a) Concerning the stomach. (b) Medicine exciting action of the stomach.

STYPTIC: (a) Contracting a blood vessel; stopping a hemorrhage by astringent action. (b) Anything that checks a hemorrhage.

SUDORIFIC: (a) Secreting or promoting the secretion of sweat. (b) Agent which produces sweating.

TAENIFUGE: An agent which expels tapeworms.

TONIC: (a) Pertaining to or characterized by tension or contraction, especially muscular tension. (b) Restoring tone. (c) A medicine that increases strength and tone.

VERMIFUGE: Agent for expelling intestinal worms.

VULNERARY: (a) Pertaining to wounds. (b) A remedy used to heal wounds.

COMMON DOSES AND EQUIVALENTS

1 teaspoonful	1 drachm
1 dessertspoonful	2 drachms
1 tablespoonful	½ fluid ounce
1 wineglassful	1½-2 fluid ounces or 3-4 tablespoonfuls
1 teacupful	4-5 fluid ounces or 8-10 tablespoonfuls

ABBREVIATIONS FOR WEIGHTS AND MEASURES

cc.	cubic centimetre(s)
dr.	drachm(s)
fl. dr.	fluid drachm(s)
fl. oz.	fluid ounce(s)
ft.	foot (feet)
g.	gramme(s)
gr.	grain(s)
in.	inch(es)
min.	minim(s)
oz.	ounce(s)
pt.	pint

TABLE OF WEIGHTS
AND MEASURES

1 grain	0.0648 grammes
1 scruple (20 grains)	1.2959 ″
1 drachm (60 grains)	3.8879 ″
1 ounce avoirdupois (437.5 grains)	28.3495 ″
1 ounce Apothecaries' or Troy (480 grains)	31.1035 ″
1 pound (7,000 grains)	453.59 ″
	or 0.4356 kilogrammes

1 minim	0.0592 millilitres
1 fluid drachm (60 minims)	3.5515 ″
1 fluid ounce (8 drachms)	28.4123 ″
1 pint (20 ounces)	0.5682 litres
1 gallon (8 pints)	4.5459 ″

1 metre	39.3701 inches
1 decimeter, 0.1 of metre	3.9370 ″
1 centimetre, 0.01 of metre	0.3970 ″
1 millimetre, 0.001 of metre	0.0397 ″

VITAMINS AND THEIR
BOTANICAL SOURCES

VITAMIN A:
Alfalfa, annatto, dandelion, lamb's quarters, okra, paprika, parsley, plankton, dulse, kelp, watercress.

VITAMIN B:
Apples, bananas, beans, beets, cabbage, carrots, cauliflower, corn, grapefruit, mushrooms, onions, oranges, peas, peanuts, potatoes, raisins, spinach, strawberries, tomatoes, turnips, wheat, yeast, bladderwrack, dulse, kelp.

Broadly speaking, I would suggest that all whole seeds contain the B vitamins.

VITAMIN C:
Fresh fruits and plants are the best sources of vitamin C. Rose hips, black currants, red currants, strawberries and practically all greens and citrus fruits. (Remember, most of the vitamin C in oranges is located in the peel and not in the juice.) Potatoes, spinach, cabbage, watercress and turnips contain relatively large amounts.

VITAMIN D:

Annatto seeds, watercress, wheat germ. I would suggest that all oil-containing seeds contain adequate amounts of vitamin D.

VITAMIN E:

Found in practically all seeds, such as alfalfa, oats, flax, sesame and wheat; in green, leafy vegetables; bladderwrack, dulse, kelp, watercress.

VITAMIN F:

Barley, coconuts, peanuts, linseed, corn, oats, olives, rice, rye, soya beans, sunflower seeds, wheat.

VITAMIN K:

Alfalfa herb, chestnut leaves, shepherd's purse.

VITAMIN P:

Apples, beets, blackberries, black currants, cabbage, carrots, cauliflower, cherries, dandelions, dock, lemons, lentils, lettuce, oranges, parsley, parsnip, peas, plums, potato, rhubarb, rose hips, mountain ash berries, spinach, turnips, tomatoes, walnuts, watercress, buckwheat, rue, paprika.

BOTANICAL SOURCES OF HORMONES

Aletris root, alfalfa herb, clover, false unicorn root, licorice, pleurisy root, sarsaparilla, yam roots and wheat. It is also believed that the following contain hormones: Alder leaves, elder flowers, garlic, linden flowers, nettles and pussy willow.

HERBAL TEAS, TISANES,
BEVERAGES AND AMBROSIALS

Contribute to the pleasantries of civilized living, aromas, fragrances, bouquets, tangs, essences, attars, pungencies and balsamics.

This flood of heavenly redolence is set free by the mere addition of hot or boiling water.

Many of these Teas have been used through the ages throughout the world for medicinal, curative, therapeutic, remedial, restorative and health-giving purposes.

ADRUE

The ground root is used for making this tea. It has a bitterish, aromatic flavor of lavender. It diffuses a feeling of warmth throughout the system and acts as a sedative.

AGRIMONY

Long used as a tea by both the English and French country

folk, especially in regions where this herb is native. Agrimony used by itself makes a pleasant, enjoyable tea. Also, it is infused with licorice root and sometimes sweetened with honey ... although the licorice itself is quite sweet and not much sweetening is required.

ANGELICA

It has a flavor resembling juniper berries and is used with juniper berries in making gin. Has a distinct flavor that resembles Chinese tea.

ANISE SEED

This is not generally used as a tea, but because of its sweet and unusual licorice-like taste, it is flavorful and pleasing.

BALM

Since time immemorial balm has been used as a brew to make a tasty, flavorful tea. The English flavored it with a few flowers of lavender. It is suggested that if a bit of rosemary is added, it gives the tea added character. Spearmint and cloves are also used to vary the flavor. It is very pleasant if iced and sweetening added. Has an odor and taste very similar to lemon.

BALM OF GILEAD

The buds make a balsamic tea with a pleasant odor and a slightly bitter taste.

BASIL

This is considered a gourmet tea of exquisite odor. It is also widely used to add flavor to other teas.

BAY LEAF

Has been used for centuries in both Greece and Italy as a tea. Also used to add flavor and aroma to other teas.

BEE BALM

This tea was used by the Oswego Indians and it is still used in parts of the New England states.

BARBERRY

Yes, this is the common Barberry and the berries make a pleasant acid drink of great utility.

BARLEY

Long known to be an excellent tea for the ill and ailing and for convalescents. It has much nutritional value.

BERGAMOT

A tea made from this plant was used by the American Indians and the early colonists. It is claimed that this tea has a "wild taste."

BETONY (Botanically *Stachys betonica*)

Back in 1676 Worlidge said, "The leaves of Chinese tea are a counterfeit of our English Betony, but far inferior to it." Antonius Musa, physician to Emperor Augustus, held Betony in such high repute he wrote a long treatise devoted to this tea. Culpeper concluded that since the Emperor did not keep fools about him, Betony surely must be a worthy tea. If a bit of dried orange peel or a clove is added, it becomes even more delicious.

BILBERRY

Also known as Whortleberry. The leaves of this plant, when dried in the shade, make a tea that in flavor, cannot be distinguished from Chinese tea. When the tea is made of the dried or fresh fruits, it has been proven particularly useful as a tonic.

BIRCH BARK

Another of the many teas used by the North American Indians. Our pioneers learned about these fine teas from them. The leaves of the birch are also used for making tea, as well as a combination of both bark and leaves. The brew exudes a sweet odor. Generally a most agreeable tea.

BONESET

Long recognized as a tea of bitter flavor. In the good old days among the early settlers, who lived under adverse conditions in log cabins with earthen floors where it was cold, damp and miserable, they found this Boneset tea invigorating and warming and the tea was generally used as a night-cap.

BURNET

Tea made from this herb, with lemon and sweetening added, was used by the French and the Indians.

CALAMINT

This has an aromatic, palatable, mint-like flavor, with a pleasant odor.

CARDAMOM

Makes a warm, grateful aromatic tea. It is made from the crushed fruits.

CASSIA PODS

This tea makes a pleasant fruit laxative.

CATNEP

In Britain this was long popular before they ever heard of Chinese tea. "Catnep is an elegant, warm, cordial aromatic" wrote Dr. Wm. Hand in 1820.

CHAMOMILE FLOWERS

Known throughout the world and long accepted as one of the most popular teas found anywhere. It is still widely used and is served throughout Europe. Loved by the Germans and the French alike. Some people drink it just as it is. Others add a bit of ginger or include a dash of fennel or a bit of honey and a slice of lemon.

CINNAMON

Has a most unusual fragrance and is widely used in the Arab countries for its ability to refresh. It is a fragrant cordial.

COMFREY

Has a sweetish taste but no odor. Improved by adding lemon. Widely accepted as a nutrient tea. Found useful and recommended for many ailments.

CORN SILK

A mild, odorless tea with a sweet flavor. A bit of licorice or ginger adds zest.

COSTMARY

Properly it is *Chrysanthemum balsamita*, but it is also known as Mint Geranium. The leaves have a lavender-like odor to them. Makes a very flavorful, minty tea. Use it carefully. Otherwise, it is apt to get too strong. The flavor is most unusual but delightful.

CUP MOSS

Makes a most invigorating and enjoyable tea if sweetened with honey. Recommended as a beverage for children.

DAMIANA

This old fragrant tea, which dates back to the days of the Spanish conquistadors, comes to us from Mexico with the highest praise. Provides a sparkling, golden brew with a most delightful aroma and an agreeable, bitterish taste. Said to encourage pleasant, amorous dreams.

DANDELION

A tea is made from the leaves of dandelions, using 1 teaspoonful to a cup. It is useful in gall bladder and rheumatic conditions.

DICTAMNUS

The flowers and foliage of this plant give off a gas which

has a strong odor and will actually ignite if a lighted match is put to it on a windless summer evening. It is referred to as Limonella by the Italians, due to the strong lemon-like scent of the leaves and the seed pods. Has a most unusual flavor that is not particularly liked by everyone.

DILL SEEDS

A tea made from dill seeds is regarded as an effective help in the case of hiccoughs. Dill seeds combined with anise seeds, chamomile and hop shoots are said to have sedative effects.

DITTANY

The leaves of this plant are dotted with aromatic oil glands. It is a native American plant which produces a most desirable tea. The pleasing aroma given off by this herb resembles a mixture of thyme and bay leaf. Exquisite.

DOG-ROSE

The fruits of the Dog-Rose, when ground up, make a sweetish and acidulous tisane. Actually, it is a good brew to give to children when it is sweetened with honey. Of course it is loaded with beneficial ascorbic acid or vitamin C.

DWARF ELDER (Botanically *Sambucus ebulus*)

The fruit of this plant makes a pleasing and invigorating tea. It is an old English favorite. With a dash of peppermint added and taken hot before retiring, it makes an excellent night-cap.

ELDER FLOWERS (Botanically *Sambucus nigras*)

Tastes sweetish at the start and then has a muscatel flavor with a touch of bitterness. Has a slight odor, but characteristic. With Peppermint added, it has long been used as a remedy against influenza.

FENNEL SEED

An agreeable tea recommended for children and the aged, when slightly sweetened with honey.

FIG

The dried figs can be soaked overnight and when hot water is added, they make a sweet, pleasing drink. It is both laxative and nutritive, and generally found to be satisfying.

FLAX SEED

Take an ounce of whole flax seed, an ounce of honey, half an ounce of licorice root and the juice of lemon. Over this pour a quart of boiling water and allow it to stand, while keeping it warm, for about four hours. Then strain off the liquor and you'll find it gratifying and palatable.

FOENUGREEK

This tea has long been used by all those who are interested in health. In fact, many people prefer it to all other teas. It is frequently used to expel phlegm. The taste and flavor remind one of celery and lovage.

GALANGAL

From a book published in 1868, "A PRACTICAL GUIDE FOR THE PERFUMER," we are told, "The Chinese prepare from it a very sweet essence, used to perfume the tea of the Emperor, and great officers of the Court." If mixed with alfalfa and strawberry leaves, it blends into a delectable brew. It is said to have been used by the Tartars.

GINGER

This is a genuine old-time favorite. Used as a stimulant and pepper-upper for chills caused by dampness or cold weather. In the West Indies it is used with a few cloves or a dash of nutmeg. The dried and sugared ginger, cut into slivers, is frequently used.

GOLDENROD

Often referred to as Blue Mountain Tea. This tea has a faint perfume. It has long been used in Pennsylvania where it was actually considered an article of commerce. When brewed it makes a delicious golden brew and has a warm anise-like flavor and fragrance.

GRINDELIA

A tea made from the herb of this plant was very largely employed in the treatment of asthmatic and bronchial affections, as well as in whooping cough and kidney diseases. It is a resinous plant with a strong scent. Has a decidedly medicinal flavor.

GROUND IVY

On the old days in Britain it was in great demand and is

still drunk in many villages. Most often it is used along with a few leaves of Melissa or Lemon Verbena, Sage, Lavender Flowers or Rosemary, with a little lemon added. It can be sweetened with honey. Licorice also improves its flavor. When using licorice, honey is not required for the licorice is sweet enough. This tea requires very little steeping.

GUARANA

The seeds of this plant are broken, roasted and then beaten into a paste and dried. The taste is astringent and bitterish, and then sweet. The odor is very much like that of chocolate. It is a popular stimulant in Brazil among the natives. They grate a small quantity into the palm of the hand and it is then swallowed and washed down with water. This vine grows in the jungles of South America. Guarana contains from two to five times as much caffeine as coffee. It is most useful as a stimulant and will keep you awake for hours, for long drives or other work that requires alertness. It can be habit-forming. It is used both hot and cold.

HAWTHORN

This well known plant, whose berries ripen in September, has been long used in botanic medicine, mainly for heart conditions, and it is considered most effective and helpful. The leaves are used in Germany where it is said to be more pleasing than Chinese green tea. Black Currant leaves, Balm and Sage are mixed with the Hawthorn leaves to make a most likeable brew.

HOP

Has a bitter taste and an aromatic flavor and odor. It is chiefly used as a bitter and is believed to improve appetite and digestion. It is usually taken warm upon retiring, as it is known to help induce sleep.

HOREHOUND

This herb has a most agreeable flavor and makes a refreshing, appetizing and healthful beverage. It is from this plant that they make the horehound ale. A nip of cayenne pepper, a dash of vinegar sweetened with honey, added to horehound tea, makes a most stimulating tea that is usually drunk hot at bedtime.

HORSEMINT

This tea is a good stimulant and like all of the mint family, it is serviceable and stimulating in various conditions. It makes a palatable beverage and it is also known to be a good diuretic and emmenagogue.

HORSEMINT (English)

The taste and odor resemble that of garden mint.

HORSETAIL

This plant is found everywhere. It does not produce flowers. Apart from its medicinal value, Horsetail is reputed as making an inviting tea. Flavored with peppermint and licorice, it is exquisite and delightful.

HYDRANGEA (Properly called *Hydrangea serrata*)

This plant is known in Japan and Korea and the leaves of this shrub are widely used as tea. The Japanese refer to it as AMA-TSJA, which in Japanese means "Tea of Heaven." The plant is widely known in cultivation in this country.

HYSSOP

Gerard states, "A decoction of Hyssope made with figges, water, honey and rue and drunken, helpeth the old cough."

JUNIPER

I believe everyone knows that the berries of the juniper plant are used in the manufacture of gin. One old highly esteemed English doctor advised to "avoid the gin and make a tea." A tea made of this plant is widely used in Bohemia.

LABRADOR

This tea has been long known to the Indians of North America, especially the Chippewas. The leaves of this plant are used to make the tea and it is claimed to be soothing, fragrant and gratifying in spite of its bitter, aromatic taste with a camphor-like odor. Has been widely used for coughs, colds, bronchial and pulmonary affections. The tea is rose-colored and tastes of the wide open spaces and has been used by Indians, frontiersmen, hunters, trappers and pioneers. A genuine outdoor tea.

LADY'S MANTLE

It is properly known as *Alchemilla vulgaris*. Use one to two teaspoons of Lady's Mantle per cup of boiling water. Allow to steep for ten minutes. Said to be of great value to women, especially during and after pregnancy. So many good things are said of this tea that I do not have space to repeat them all here.

LANTANA

Properly known as *Lantana camara*. It is a semi-tropical

230

North American plant, with interesting multicolored flowers. It is unusual but all colors are frequently found simultaneously in a single cluster. The tea is widely used but mainly by the natives where the shrub is found. It has a strong flavor and odor and is not popular, except among the natives.

LAVENDER

Has a strong, fragrant odor that is quite characteristic of the plant. It is not often used as a tea in itself because of its rather strong flavor. It is generally mixed with other herbs. The tea is usually made from the flowers.

LEMON GRASS

Properly known as *Cymbopogon shaenanthus*, this is the plant with the lemon-scented foliage. Cultivated in India for centuries. The tea made from this plant is esteemed mainly by the people of the West Indies, where it has long been regarded as a delectable brew. Because it is so highly praised by those who know it, it is well worth trying. It is best served piping hot.

LEMON VERBENA

To obtain the highest pleasure from the drinking of regular Chinese tea, add a few leaves of Lemon Verbena. If you like it sweet, add a teaspoon of honey and, as one authority claims, "No beverage can compare with it." When the leaves of this plant are rubbed they give off a distinct lemon-like odor and the taste resembles that of lemon.

LICORICE

The best tea is made from the ground pieces of root, not the woody sticks. The plants yield a substance known as glycyrrhiza, which is said to be 50 times sweeter than cane sugar. It is a great thirst quencher. May be used either hot or cold. It is used by itself and also with other teas.

LIME FRUIT

The juice of this fruit taken as is or with honey makes a most enjoyable tea. Often used with alcoholic beverages. One of the earliest known antiscorbutics.

LINDEN

Long a favorite in Europe and served in many European eating establishments. The tea has a bouquet similar to that of Sweet Jasmine. Best served with lemon, if iced. If taken before retiring, hot, it induces pleasant sleep and is most relaxing.

LIPPIA

Properly known as *Lippia dulcis*. It has an agreeable, aromatic taste and odor. Recognized as an excellent remedy for coughs, colds, whooping cough and bronchial affection.

LOVAGE

A tisane made from lovage tastes actually more like a broth than a tea. It is one of the few teas that can be drunk or taken with salt, if preferred, instead of sugar or honey. It is claimed to have the effect of an internal bath and thus acts as a deodorant.

MARJORAM

The tea is made from the herbs and leaves. It has an aromatic and agreeable flavor. Regarded as a tonic and a stimulant.

MUGWORT

Still used as a common tea in Cornwall. Sometimes mint or pennyroyal is added, and sweetened with honey. It should not be steeped very long. It is recommended for old people because of its mildness.

MULBERRY

The fruit of the Mulberry, when squeezed and the juice extracted, forms a grateful drink for convalescents and is said to check the thirst and cool the blood. I have often made a tea of the fruit by pouring hot water over them.

NETTLE

The herb makes a nice botanic beer. It is also used as a medicine in nettle rash. The infusion of 1 oz. either herb or seed to 1 pt. of boiling water is taken in wineglassful doses. Said to have been introduced into England by the Roman invaders. It is made like Chinese tea, sweetened and flavored with lemon to taste. It is also often mixed with Chinese Tea: 1 part nettles to 3 parts tea.

OLD ENGLISH

From a book on Domestic Economy, 1839: "Take of Hawthorn leaves, dried, 2 parts; Sage and Balm, 2 parts. Mix these well together and they will make an excellent and pleasant tea, particularly wholesome for people who must avoid stimulating beverages."

PARAGUAY

It is commonly known as Yerba or Yerba Mate. To South

Americans, Yerba is the only drink. It is also widely used in North America. It definitely has stimulating properties, without the harmful effects of tea or coffee. It is used as a green leaf tea, and there is also a tea made from the bark and the stems and the leaves, all ground up into a powder. Most South Americans prefer this powder and they like it real strong.

PARSLEY

A highly nutritious tea. It is often mixed with alfalfa, yellow dock root and watercress.

PEACH

The leaves of the Peach tree are used by the Chinese in making a tea, which they claim has many medicinal uses; specifically for irritation and congestion of the gastric surfaces, as well as coughs, whooping cough and chronic bronchitis. It is taken in small quantities.

PENNYROYAL

A stimulating beverage. The taste and odor are distinctly minty, but it still retains its own characteristics. It is sometimes mixed with Lavender flowers. Most frequently taken hot upon retiring.

PEPPERMINT

Next to Chinese tea I would suggest that Peppermint tea is one of the most widely used of all herb teas. It deservedly earns the high esteem in which it is held. It can be given freely to children, which cannot be done with either Chinese tea or coffee or most other beverages. Peppermint tea also forms the basis of many other herb teas. It is often mixed with alfalfa, clover flowers, linden flowers, chamomile, licorice, strawberry leaves, raspberry leaves and others.

PERSIMMON

The leaves of the Persimmon make a most exquisite tea. Claimed to be better than Chinese tea and it is rich in vitamin C.

PIPSISSEWA

Properly known as *Chimaphila umbellata*. Another one of the many Indian teas that was used by the early fur traders and pioneers. Gives off a most delightful reddish color with a rich flavor, but it is definitely bitterish. Honey or licorice will sweeten it.

POMEGRANATE

The fruit and the rind can be used in making tea. This is one of the oldest known fruits on earth. Said to be a specific for the removal of tape worm.

POTENTILLA

From this plant is made a popular tea known as Five Finger Tea. It is used mainly by the folks living in the Ozarks, Arkansas, Kentucky and Tennessee. The plant is a sprawling wayside weed which resembles wild Strawberry.

PRUNE

The juice of the prune makes a most delightful and refreshing tea, and it is also a safe, sure laxative. The dried fruit is soaked for 24 to 48 hours in water and the resulting juice may then be drunk cold or hot.

QUINCE

The fruit of the Quince tree can be made into a most inviting, delicious tea. The taste, aroma and odor are entirely distinctive. Use with honey or licorice. It is hard to surpass.

RASPBERRY LEAF

Used for centuries in Europe and considered especially useful for pregnant women. Widely esteemed and used. Found in many of the herbal tea blends.

RED CLOVER FLOWERS

More widely used than most people realize. Said to be useful in the treatment of cancer. Has a mild, delicate flavor. Once very popular and its popularity is coming back. Sweeten with honey. Try it with some Chamomile flowers, too. Serve it hot or cold.

ROSEMARY

Was used many hundreds of years ago by the Arabian physicians, who were probably the first to recommend this fragrant herb as a tea. Said to clear up many cases of headache. If Lavender flowers, a bit of lemon and honey are added, it becomes most inviting and captivating.

SAGE

Care must be taken not to make the brew too strong. Heavenly if sweetened with maple syrup. Sometimes flavored with a dash of orange or lemon, or a pinch of mace or cinnamon. It is also exquisite mixed with Melissa. It is claimed that the Chinese preferred Sage Tea to their own native tea and would trade twice the quantity of their choicest tea for it.

ST. JOHN'S BREAD

The pods of this plant, when ground up, make a sweet, chocolate-flavored brew. It is considered highly nutritive and is claimed to improve the voice. It requires no sweetening as the pods themselves are quite sweet.

SARSAPARILLA

Here is a suggested brew. Use 1 part Sarsaparilla, 1 part Sassafras, 1/2 part Snakeroot, and allow the tea to brew for at least five minutes. Keep the lid on the pot. Maple syrup is ideal for sweetening.

SASSAFRAS

The bark of the root ground to a powder is generally used for this tea. Only a quarter of a teaspoonful is required to make a cup. The leaves can also be used but I have found the root of the bark preferable. It has definite stimulating qualities.

SENNA

It has a sweet but sickly flavor. The odor is distinctly tea-like. It is generally combined with other aromatic and stimulating herbs to modify its griping effects. But it has been used successfully for centuries as a laxative and a cathartic. Here is a suggested infusion: Senna leaves 2 ozs., Ginger 1 dr., boiling water 1 pt. Let it stand for an hour, strain through muslin and take in wineglassful doses.

SLIPPERY ELM

Ground Slippery Elm bark, when boiled and strained and then flavored with lemon juice and honey, not only makes a delicious tea but something that is most nutritious, palatable and refreshing. Considered an excellent food or beverage for invalids or children.

SLOE BERRY

In an old Encyclopedia it is claimed that the young, tender leaves afford the best substitute for the foreign teas. Properly it is known as *Viburnum prunifolium*. The berries are exceptionally sweet.

SPEARMINT

Similar in its flavor and properties to Peppermint. Slightly milder and more fragrant. Useful as a beverage for children.

SPEEDWELL

Has a bitter astringent taste, with a slight fragrance. Used in Europe as a substitute for Chinese tea and thought by some to be equal or superior to it. One authority claims "that it forms a more grateful beverage than the Chinese tea."

SUMACH BERRIES

The Ojibway Indians used the berries of this plant to make a cooling drink for summer and they boiled it hot for the winter. It has a pleasant acid flavor.

SUMMER SAVORY

It has an aromatic piquancy and taste, recalling thyme and marjoram, but distinctive. Said to be one of the most stimulating of herb teas.

SWEET BAY

Down in the Everglades the Seminoles use the leaves of this plant for making a tea which they highly prize as a wholesome beverage.

SWEET CICELY

Has a sweet anise-like taste or flavor. Used as a tonic and stimulant tea and is also useful in coughs and flatulence.

TEA TREE

It is properly known as *Leptospermum scoparium*. The crew of Captain Cook's ship, as well as other early navigators, used the leaves of this tree for making tea. It is still used in New Zealand and Australia. Usually found only in the far East.

TEA (*Camellia sinensis*)

No list of teas would actually be complete without listing what the world recognizes as the TRUE tea, which is also known as *Thea chinensis* and *Camellia theifera*. It is an evergreen shrub that grows in the hills of China, India, Ceylon and perhaps other parts of the world. The leaf buds, together with two or three young leaves, are collected and allowed to wither. They are then rolled and fermented, and the color changes from green to black. Part of the tannin is oxidized and traces of volatile oil are produced. Green tea is obtained by

239

drying over a fire and in this way the tannin is not oxidized and the leaves retain their green color. The principal constituents are caffeine and tannin.

THYME

Brew this the same way as you would Chinese tea. This brew gives off its best flavor when iced and served with lemon. Makes an excellent brew along with alfalfa, strawberry, red clover, raspberry, sassafras, licorice and others. Said to be a warming tea for the aged.

VALERIAN

Has a sweetish, bitter taste and a characteristic odor. Taken in wineglassful doses it allays pain and promotes sleep. It is of benefit to the nerves without any narcotic effects.

VERBASCUM

It is valuable when hoarse or when losing one's voice, particularly for those who speak or sing, or when having difficulty in breathing. It can be used for children and old people as well.

VERVAIN

Properly known as *Verbena officinalis*. This tea is a sedative and stimulates the production of bile. Used in nervous exhaustion and as a sedative and digestive. It is slightly bitter and soothing. Use one teaspoon of Vervain per cup. Allow to steep for only five minutes. It is said to clear the eyes and the sight.

WILD MARJORAM

Properly it is known as *Origanum vulgare*. An old book on medical botany states, "The leaves of Wild Marjoram, when dried, are used instead of tea, and are said to be exceedingly grateful." Wild Marjoram tea has a flavor that resembles a blend of thyme, rosemary and sage.

WINTERGREEN

This tea is rose-colored and possesses its own natural sweet flavor. No sweetening agent need be added. The tea is unusual in that it leaves a most pleasant lingering after-taste. Said to be a very valuable remedy in the treatment of rheumatism. Of benefit to infants who have trouble with their stomachs.

WOODRUFF

By simply steeping the dried leaves to the desired strength, you will find a most fragrant and palatable brew. The herb acquires a vanilla-like aroma when it is dried. Said to be one of the most agreeable and delightful of all herb teas. Used to flavor candies, wine and liquors. Tastes like coumarine and when dried, it smells just like new-mown hay.

YARROW

Distinctly used as a medicinal brew by the old herbal practitioners. Used as a beverage by Swiss mountaineers. I know of no one else who uses it. It has an insipid flavor and a feeble odor. However, combined with elder flowers, peppermint and honey, it makes an agreeable, delectable brew. Said to be of value for influenza and colds.

USING HERBAL TEAS

The merits of teas in herbalism are many. If they did nothing else but make it possible to avoid the use of black tea, coffee, postum and other beverages that are made from burnt or highly heated and treated substances, they would contribute greatly to the health of the population. It is an established fact that all burnt substances are carcinogenic.

Black teas are subjected to high heat and fermentation as well as other treatments. Thus, the use of herbal teas will eliminate the dangers in that direction. Apart from this, herb teas in variety would prevent the accumulation of various components as well as the resulting deficiencies that create an imbalance in the human body.

Actually, tea is an infusion of an herb in hot water. In many cases the nutrients or food values contained within the herb are found in the resulting tea. Therefore, instead of suffering ill or harm from regular tea and other burnt substances like coffee and postum, one would receive benefits from drinking herb tea.

It is suggested that when tea is brewed it be drunk immediately or within a few minutes after brewing. Leaving it brew, stew or sit for a long time does not enhance its pleasantness or nutritional value. However, there are some exceptions to this rule.

Where milk or a sweetening is desired, by all means use it; but to obtain the best flavor and pleasure from tea, it is best without either.

I was once a heavy user of tea and, to a lesser degree, of coffee. I used to drink from eight to twelve cups of tea every single day. I found that it wasn't that I enjoyed the tea-drinking so much, but the fact that I enjoyed the moments or hours of pleasantness spent over a cup of tea with loved ones, friends and acquaintances.

Then, quite by accident, I learned of the beauty, the fragrance and the pleasantness of herb teas and have been a confirmed herb tea drinker since that day.

Among the other benefits of herb teas are flavor, aroma, bouquet, nutrients and healing qualities.

It is not suggested that any or all herb teas are necessarily suited for drinking after or with meals, or as a daily routine.

I have learned that you can offer herb teas to conventional tea and coffee drinkers and most will enjoy them and often become converted to the use of these flavorful, pleasant tisanes.

Admittedly, serving the proper tea at the right time and knowing how to prepare it is in itself an art worth acquiring.

Now I do not believe that any general rule of thumb can be followed. The method generally given is to use one teaspoonful of tea per cup and then another teaspoonful for the pot. My experience with herb teas does not indicate this rule to be valid. There are many teas where one teaspoonful per cup would be much too much. For example, with sassafras, licorice or sage, a teaspoonful per cup would be over-powering. Therefore, I would suggest that with every different brew you try different strengths and then decide the amount to be used in each case.

It is generally suggested that boiling water be used, but strange to relate, I have learned that you can use water hot,

243

without being boiled, and get results that are even better. Furthermore, in this way you do not harm most of the nutrients found in the herbs.

I would set five minutes as the maximum for the steeping and then pour.

Good spring or well water is best. Try to avoid chlorinated, fluorinated or otherwise chemically treated water. You just cannot get good results from water that contains added chemicals; although I do know that many people use strong herb teas to disguise the taste of the heavily chemicalized water.

The preferred pot is of course an earthenware pot. Porcelain pots are used and so are enamel pots. I would consider them fair. I have also seen many iron pots. To any of these I do not object, but one pot that I would definitely advise avoiding is an aluminum pot. Now I have no prejudice against aluminum except that it should never be used in or along with food of any kind.

Do not use herb teas that have to be filtered through a sack. That is, don't use herb teas in paper or cloth bags. You will never get the true bouquet or aroma or flavor from them.

GATHER YOUR OWN HERBS

I felt that this book would be incomplete if it did not include a section on the gathering and preservation of herbs.

In this day and age in America the gathering and drying of herbs has become a lost art, although at no time did it ever reach the perfection that it achieved in Asia and Europe.

Therefore, I felt the best contribution I could make to those of you who would like to gather and dry your own herbs would be to call upon an eminent ranking authority on the subject, Thomas Green, as contained in Volume One of his Universal Herbal (1820).

GENERAL RULES
FOR
GATHERING AND PRESERVING HERBS,

ROOTS, BARK, SEEDS, AND FLOWERS;

Together With the Methods of Making Such Preparations From Them, as May Best Retain Their Virtues, or Be Most Useful to be Kept in Families.

The intention of the author is, to inform those who live in the country, and are desirous of being useful to their families and friends, or charitable to the poor in relieving their disorders, of the virtues of those plants which grow wild about them; that they may be able to supply the necessary assistance, in places where apothecaries are not at hand, without putting themselves to the expense of costly medicines, when the common herbs, that may be had for gathering, will answer the same purpose. However, as there are cases wherein more help may be obtained from foreign drugs, than from any thing produced at home, an account of those roots, barks, seeds, gums, and other vegetable productions, kept by the druggists and apothecaries, is added, together with their virtues, and those of the several trees and plants from which they are obtained.

The plants are alphabetically arranged, according to their English names, that they may be the more readily found. With regard to the virtues of plants, too many have been attributed to most of them, but here their real virtues only, as ascertained by the experience of the best judges, are introduced, and placed in the most conspicuous light.

Nature has, in this country, as well as in all others, provided, in the herbs of its own growth, the remedies for the several diseases to which it is most subject; and although the addition of what is brought from abroad, should not be supposed superfluous, there is no occasion that it should cause the other to be neglected. This neglect has been the consequence of the too great respect shewn to them; which, with the present universal use of chemical preparations, has almost driven the whole of Galenical medicine out of our minds.

To restore this more safe, more gentle, and often more efficacious part of medicine to its natural credit, has been one great intent in writing this treatise; and it is the more necessary for the service of those, who are intended most to be directed in this matter, since this is much less dangerous than the other; for in most instances it is hard to say that this is dangerous at all.

The apothecaries are apt, in their unfeeling mockery, to say, that they are obliged to the good persons who give medicines to their sick neighbours, for a great deal of their business; for out of little disorders they make great ones. This may be the case *where their shops supply the means;* for chemical medicines, and some of the drugs brought from abroad, are not to be trusted with those who have not great experience; but there will be no danger of this kind, when the fields afford the supply. This is the medicine of nature, and as it is more efficacious in most cases, it is more safe in all. If opium may be dangerous in an unexperienced hand, the person who will give in its place a syrup of the wild lettuce, (a plant not known in common practice at this time, but recommended from experience in this treatise) will find that it will ease pain, and that it will cause sleep, in the manner of that foreign drug, but will never find any ill consequences from it: and the same might be said in many other instances.

As the descriptions in this work very readily distinguish what are the real plants that should be used, the great care will remain, in what manner to gather and preserve, and in what manner to give them; it will be useful to add directions upon those heads. As to the *former,* it should be perfectly understood, because a great deal depends upon it; the *latter* cannot easily be mistaken.

Having displaced the drugs brought from abroad in a great measure from charitable practice, every person who has the spirit of true benevolence, should keep a kind of druggist's shop, which should be supplied from the neighbouring fields,

247

and from their own gardens. There is no reason the drugs should not be as well preserved, and as carefully laid up, as if the product of a different climate, though the use of the fresh plants will in general be best when they can be had.

As there are some which will not retain their virtues in a dried state, and can be met with only during a small part of the year; it will be proper to add the best methods of preserving these in some way, according to the apothecaries' manner; with the method of making the preparations from them for ready service, which will be sufficient to lead to the perfect use of the medicines of our own growth; and it will be found upon experience, that those who sufficiently know how to make a proper use of these, need seldom have recourse to any others.

Concerning the Methods of Collecting and Preserving Plants, and Parts of them, for use.

The virtues of different plants residing principally in certain parts of them, and those differing according to the nature of the herb, these several parts are to be selected, and the rest left; and these are in some to be used fresh, and just gathered; in others, either necessity, or the natural preference, make it proper to dry and preserve them.

In some only the leaves are to be used; in others, the whole plant cut from the root; in others, the flowers only; in others, the fruits; in others, the seeds; in some, the roots; and of some trees, the barks; some, the woods; and only the excrescences of others; while some vegetables are to be used entire, whether fresh gathered, or dried and preserved. Of all these, instances will be given in great number in the following pages, and the matter will be specified under each article, as the part of the plant to be used will always be named; and it will be added whether it be fresh, or best or necessarily dried or otherwise preserved; but it will be proper in this place to enter into full examination of this matter, to save unnecessary repetitions under the several particular articles.

The whole of most plants native of our country, dies off in winter, except the root; and in many, that perishes also, leaving the species to be renewed from the fallen seeds. When the whole plant dies, the root is seldom of any virtue; but when the root remains many years, and sends up new shoots in the spring, it commonly has great virtue. This may be a general rule: for there is very little to be expected in the roots of annual plants; their seeds, for the most part, contain their greatest virtues.

In others, the root lives through the winter, and there arise from it large leaves in the spring, before the stalk appears. These are to be distinguished from those which afterwards grow on the stalk, for they are more juicy, and for many purposes much better. In the same manner, some plants, from their seeds dropped in autumn, produce a root and leaves which stand all the winter, and the stalk does not rise till the succeeding spring. These are of the nature of those leaves, which rise from the root of other plants before the stalks in spring; and are in the same manner to be distinguished from those which grow upon the stalks; they have the full nourishment from the root, whereas the others are starved by the growth of the stalk and its branches, and the preparations made by nature for the flowers and seeds; which are the great purpose of nature, as they are to continue the plant.

For this reason, when the leaves of any plant are said to be the part fittest for use, they are not to be taken from the stalk, but these large ones growing from the root are to be chosen; and these where there is no stalk, if that can be; for then only they are fullest of juice, and have their complete virtue; the stalk running away with the nourishment from them. This is so

249

much done in some plants, that although the leaves growing from the root were very vigorous before the stalk grew up, they die and wither as it rises.

When the juice of the leaves of any plant is required, these are the leaves from which it is to be pressed: when they are ordered in decoction, notice is always taken in this work, whether they be best fresh or dried; if fresh, they should be just gathered for the occasion; they should be cut up close from the root, and only shook clean, not washed; for in many, that carries off a part of the virtue: they are to be cut into the pot. If they are to be dried, the same caution is to be used; and they are best dried by spreading them upon the floor of the room, with the windows open, often turning them. When thoroughly dried, they should be put up in a drawer, pressing them close down, and covered with paper. When the entire plant is to be used except the root, care is to be taken that it be gathered at a proper season. Nature, in the whole growth of plants, tends to the production of their flowers and seeds, but when they are ripe, the rest begins to decay, having done its duty; so that the time when the entire plant is in its most full perfection, is when it is in the bud; when the heads are formed for flowering, but not a single flower has yet disclosed itself: this is the exact time.

When herbs are to be used fresh, it is best not to take them entire, but only to cut off the tops; three or four inches long, if for infusion, and if for other purposes, less: if they are to be beaten up with sugar, they should be only an inch, or less: just as far as they are fresh and tender. The tops of the plant thus gathered, are always preferable to the whole plant for immediate use.

When the entire herb is to be dried, the season for gathering is to be as just described, when the flowers are budding; and the time of the day must be when the morning dew is dried away. This is a very material circumstance, for if they be cut wet with the dew, herbs will not dry well, and if they be cut at noon-day, when the sun has made the leaves flag, they will not have their full power.

Care must also be taken to cut them in a dry day; for the wet of rain will do as much harm as that of dew.

When the herbs are thus gathered, they are to be looked over, the decayed leaves to be picked off, and the dead ends of the stalks cut away: they are then to be tied up in small bunches, (the smaller the better,) and hung upon lines drawn across a room, where the windows and doors are kept open in good weather; the bunches are to be half a foot asunder, and they are to hang till perfectly dry. They are then to be taken softly down, without shaking off the buds of the flowers, and laid evenly in a drawer, pressing them down, and covering them with paper. They are thus ready for infusions and decoctions, and are better for distillation than when fresh.

The flowers of plants are principally used fresh, though several particular kinds retain their virtue very well dried; they are on these different occasions to be treated differently.

Lavender flowers, and those of stoecha, keep very well; they are therefore to be preserved dry; the lavender flowers are to be stripped off the stalks, husk and all together, and spread upon the floor of a room to dry. The stoechas flowers are to be preserved in the whole head; this is to be cut off from the top of the stalk, and dried in the same manner: when dry, they are to be kept as the herbs.

When rosemary flowers are dried, they are generally taken with some of the leaves about them; and this is very right, for the leaves retain more virtue than the flowers. Some dry borage, bugloss, and cowslips, but they retain very little virtue in that condition. Rose-buds are to be dried, and to this purpose, their white heads are to be cut off; and the full-blown flowers may be preserved in the same manner. The red rose is always meant, when we speak of the dried flowers.

For the rest of the flowers used in medicine, they are best fresh; but as they remain only a small part of the year in that state, the method is to preserve them in the form of syrups and conserves. Such as the syrup of cloves and poppies, the conserves of cowslips, and the like. Of these, a short general account shall be subjoined, that nothing may be wanting to make this work as useful for families as the nature of it will admit.

Among the fruits of plants, several are to be used fresh, as the hip for conserve, and the quince, mulberry, and black currant; from the juices of which, syrups are made. As to those which are to be dried, as the juniper berries, the bay berries, and the like, they are only to be gathered when just ripening, not when quite mellow, and spread upon a table or floor, often turning them till they are dry. But of these we use very few of our own growth; most of the fruits used in medicine are brought from abroad, and must be purchased of the druggist or apothecary.

With respect to the seeds and plants, it is otherwise: many of them are of our own growth, and nothing is so easy as to preserve them. These are all to be used dry; but nature has in manner dried them to our hands: for they are not to be gathered till perfectly ripe, and then they need very little farther care. They are only to be spread for three or four days upon a clean floor, where the air has free passage, but where the sun does not come; and they are then ready to be put up.

The seeds used in medicine, may be referred to three general kinds. They either grow in naked heads or umbels, as in fennel, parsley, and the like; or in pods, as in mustard and cresses; or in large fleshy fruits, as in melon and cucumbers. In each case they must be left upon the plant till perfectly ripe; then they are only to be shook from the heads upon the floor, or if in pods, a smart stroke or two of the plant upon the floor, when they are thoroughly ripe, will dislodge them. In the other case, the fruit must be cut open, and they must be taken out from among the wet matter, separated from the membranes that are about them, and spread upon a table, in a dry place, where they must be often turned and rubbed as they grow dry, that in the end they may be perfectly dry and clean.

Among the roots, a great many are to be used fresh, but a greater number are best dried. The black and white briony, the arum, and some others, lose all their virtues in drying; and many that retain some, yet lose the greater part of it: there are others which are excellent, both fresh and dried, as the marshmallow and some more.

As to the few which lose their virtue entirely in drying, it will be best to keep some of them always in the garden, that they may be taken up as they are wanted. The others are to be managed according to their several natures, and they do a great deal towards furnishing the druggist's shop, which should be filled with medicines, the produce of our own country.

The best season for gathering roots for drying, is in the early part of the spring; what nature does for plants when they are just going to flower, she does for roots when the leaves are just going to bud; the juices are rich, fresh, and full, and the virtue is strongest in them at this season; therefore they are to be then taken up.

In the end of February and the beginning of March, the ground should be searched for the first budding of leaves, and the roots taken up. They are to be wiped clean, not washed; and, according to their several natures, prepared for drying.

Some are full of mucilaginous juice, as marshmallow, and above all other roots, the squill, and in some degree many others of that kind; these must be cut into thin slices crosswise, and they will dry best if laid upon a hair-cloth stretched across a frame. They must be frequently turned, and be very thoroughly dry before they are put up, else they will become mouldy; but, rightly prepared, they keep very well.

Other roots have juices that evaporate more easily. These have the virtue either throughout the whole substance, or only in the outer part, and they are to be prepared accordingly. When roots are of one uniform substance, they generally have the virtue equal, or nearly so, in all parts. These should be split open lengthwise, first cutting off the head, and the little end; or if considerably thick, they may be quartered; when this is done, they are to be strung upon a line, by drawing a needle, threaded with a small twine, through their thickest part, and they are then to be hung up to dry in the manner of the herbs; the line being stretched across a room, the doors and windows of which are to be kept open in good weather.

When roots consist of a sort of thick rind, or fleshy substance within the rind, and a hard sticky part in the middle, this fleshy substance under it possesses all the virtues; the hard inner substance having none: in this case, the root is to be split longwise as before, and the hard woody part is to be taken out and thrown away: the rest is to be strung, as before described, and dried in the same manner.

When roots consist of fibres, these are generally connected

254

to a head, if it be ever so small, and the best method is to split this in two, and then string up the separate parts for drying.

It is needless to enumerate the examples of the several kinds of roots here; they follow in their places: but if charitable people would, on first looking over this book to see what are most useful, order their gardener to take out of his ground, and to seek in the fields the several roots there mentioned, and see them dried and preserved according to these directions, they would be possessed of a set of drugs of a new kind indeed; but they would save the price of many brought from other countries, and might be used with less danger.

The barks of trees make but a small part of the English drugs, and most of them are best fresh; but such as will preserve and retain their virtues dried, are very easily prepared that way: nothing more is required than to cut them up in the same manner as the roots. When they are dry, they are to be put up as the others, and they will keep ever so long; but in all this time they are for the most part losing their virtues.

It may be prudent to preserve drugs brought from abroad a great while, because of their price; but as these cost only the trouble of gathering and preserving them, I would advise that the whole shop be renewed every year; what is left of the old parcel of every kind, being thrown away as the fresh one is collected in its season.

The place for keeping these should be a dry room, neither damp nor hot; and they should now and then be looked at, to see that they are in order; that they do not grow mouldy, or smell musty, through damp, or become lighter, and lose their virtue by too much heat.

It may be proper just to mention, that the woods which

we use are best kept in the block, and shaved off as they are wanted; for being kept in shavings, they lose their virtue: and in the same manner as to the foreign woods, it is best to keep a block of sassafras, and of lignum vitae, in the house, and cut them as they are wanted.

As to the excrescences, such as galls of the oak, and the burr from the wild briar, they are naturally so dry, that they only require to be exposed a few days to the air upon a table; and then they may be put up with safety, and will keep a long time.

Lastly, the funguses, such as Jew's-ears, and the like, are to be gathered when they are full grown, and strung upon a line; they must dry leisurely, or else they spoil: they must be very well dried before they are put up, else they will grow mouldy in damp weather; and if once that happen, no art can recover their virtues.

Thus may a druggist's shop of a new kind be filled, and it will consist of as many articles as those which receive their furniture from abroad; and there will be this advantage in having every thing ready; that when custom has made the virtues of the several things familiar, any person may do from his judgment as the physician in his prescription — mix several things of like virtue together, and not depend upon the virtues of any one singly, when the case requires something of power. These roots and barks powdered, will make as handsome and as efficacious boluses and mixtures as any furnished by the apothecary.

Concerning the Various Methods of Preparing Simples for Present Use.

256

There is no form of medicines sent from the apothecary, which may not be prepared from the herbs of our own growth, in the same manner as from foreign drugs. Electuaries may be made with the powders of these barks, roots, and seeds, with conserves of flowers, and of the tops of fresh herbs; and syrups, made from their juices and infusions; the manner of making which is very simple, and shall be subjoined to this chapter, that all may be understood before we enter on the book itself: and in the same manner their boluses may be made, which are only some of these powders mixed up with syrup: and their draughts and juleps, which are made from the distilled waters of these herbs, with spirit, or without these, syrups being added and the tinctures of the roots and barks; the method of making which shall be also annexed in a familiar manner.

But beside these several forms of giving them, there are others much more simple, easy, and ready, and these are generally more efficacious. We shall arrange these under three kinds; juices, infusions, and decoctions. These are the forms of giving the medicines most frequently mentioned in the course of the work, and there is less trouble in them than in the others. They are not indeed contrived for show, nor would they answer the purpose of the apothecary, for his profits would be small upon them; but when the design is only to do good, they are most to be chosen of any.

Juices are to be expressed from leaves or roots; and in order to do this, they are to be first beaten in a mortar. There is no form whatever in which herbs have so much effect, and yet this is in a manner unknown in the common practice of physic.

These are to be obtainied in some plants from the entire herb, as in watercresses, brooklime, and others that have juicy stalks; in others the leaves are to be used, as in nettles, and the like, where the stalk is dry, and yields nothing, but is

257

troublesome in the preparation. When the juice of a root is to be had, it must be fresh taken up, and thoroughly beaten. A marble mortar and wooden pestle serve best for this purpose, for any thing of metal is improper: many plants would take a tincture from it, and the juice would be so impregnated with it, as to become a different medicine, and probably very improper in the case in which it was about to be given.

As these juices have sometimes an ill taste, and as some of them are apt to be cold upon the stomach, or otherwise to disagree with it, there are methods to be used to make them sit better upon it; and in some cases these increase their virtues.

When the thick juice, fresh drawn, is too coarse for the person's stomach, it may be suffered to settle and grow clear: a little sugar may be added also in beating the herb, and in many cases, as in those juices given for the scurvy, the juice of a Seville orange may be added, which will greatly improve the flavour.

To the roots it is often proper to add a little white wine in the bruising, and they will operate the better for it. Thus, for instance, the juice of the flower-de-luce root will not stay upon many stomachs alone; but with a little white wine added in the bruising, all becomes easy, and its effects are not the less for the addition. The same addition may be made to some of the colder herbs; and if a little sugar, and, upon occasion, a few grains of powdered ginger, be added, there will be scarce any fear of the medicine disagreeing with the stomach, and its effects will be the same as if it had been bruised and pressed alone.

Infusions are naturally to be mentioned after the juices, for they are in many cases used to supply their place. Juices can only be obtained from fresh plants, and there are times of the year when the plants are not to be had in that state. Recourse is then to be had to the shop, instead of the field; the plant whose juice cannot be had, is there to be found dried and preserved; and if that has been done according to the preceding directions, it retains a great part of its virtues: in this case it is to be cut to pieces, and hot water being poured upon it, extracts so much of its qualities, as to stand in the place of the other. Often, indeed, the virtues are the same, in some plants they are greatest from the infusion; but then some others lose so much in drying, that an infusion scarce has anything. But it is not only as a help in the place of the other, that this preparation is to be used, for infusions are very proper from many fresh herbs; and are of great virtue from many dry ones, of which, when fresh, the juice would have been worth little.

Infusions are the fittest forms for those herbs whose qualities are light, and whose virtue is easily extracted: in this case, hot water poured upon them takes up enough of their virtue, and none is lost in the operation; others require to be boiled in the water. From these are thus made what we call decoctions: and as these last would not give their virtues in infusion, so the others would lose it all in the boiling; it would go off with the vapour. We know very well, that the distilled water of any herb is only the vapour of the boiled herb caught by proper vessels, and condensed to water: therefore, whether it be caught or let to fly away, all that virtue must be lost in boiling. It is from this, that some plants are fit for decoctions, and some for infusions. There are some which, if distilled, give no virtue to the water; and those are fit for decoctions, which will retain all their virtue, as bistort, and tormentil roots, and the like. On the contrary, an infusion of mint, or pennyroyal, is of a strong taste, and excellent virtue; whereas a decoction of these herbs is disagreeable, or good for nothing.

There are herbs also, which have so little juice that it would be impossible to get it out; and others, whose virtue lies in the husks and buds, and this would be lost in the operation. An infusion of these is the right way of giving them. Thus, mother of thyme is a dry little herb, from which it would be hard to get any juice, and when gotten, it would possess very little of its virtues; but an infusion of mother of thyme possesses it entirely.

Infusions are of two kinds. They are either prepared in quantity, to be drank cold; or they are drank as they are made, in the manner of tea. This last method is the best, but people will not be prevailed upon to do it, unless the taste of the herb be agreeable; for the flavour is much stronger hot than it is cold.

Infusions in the manner of tea, are to be made just as tea, and drank with a little sugar; the others are to be made in this manner:

A stone jar is to be fitted with a close cover; the herb, whether fresh or dried, is to be cut to pieces; and when the jar has been scalded out with hot water, it is to be put in: boiling water is then to be poured upon it, and the top is to be fixed on: it is thus to stand four, five, or six hours, or a whole night, according to the nature of the ingredient, and then to be poured off clear.

It is impossible to direct the quantity in general for these infusions, because much more of some plants is required than of others: for the most part, three quarters of an ounce of a dried plant, or two ounces of the fresh gathered. The best rule is, to suit it to the patient's strength and palate. It is intended not to be disagreeable, and to have as much virtue of the herb as is necessary: this is only to be known in each kind by trial; and the virtue may be heightened, as well as the flavour mended, by several additions. Of these, sugar and a little white wine are the most familiar, but lemon juice is often very serviceable, as we find in sage tea; and a few drops of oil of vitriol give colour and strength to tincture of roses. Salt of tartar makes many infusions stronger also than they would be, but it gives them a very disagreeable taste. It is therefore fit only for such as are to be taken at one draught, not for such as are to be swallowed in large quantities time after time.

Among the herbs that yield their virtues most commodiously by infusion, may be accounted many of those which are pectoral, and good in coughs, as coltsfoot, ground-ivy and the like: the light and aromatic, good in nervous disorders, as mother of thyme, balm, and the like: the bitter are also excellent in infusion, but very disagreeable in decoction; thus boiling water poured upon Roman wormwood, gentian root, and orange peel, makes a very excellent bitter. It need only stand till the liquor is cold, and may be then poured off for use.

It is often proper to add some purging ingredient to this bitter infusion; and a little fresh polypody root excellently answers that purpose, without spoiling the taste of the medicine.

Several of the purging plants also do very well in infusion, as purging flax, and the like; and the fresh root of polypody alone is a very good one: a little lemon-juice added to the last named infusion does no harm; and it takes off what is disagreeable in the taste, in the same manner as it does from an infusion of senna.

Thus we see what a great number of purposes may be answered by infusions, and they are the most familiar of all preparations. Nothing is required, but pouring some boiling water upon the plants fresh or dried, as already directed, and pouring it off again when cold.

261

Decoctions are contrived to answer the purpose of infusions, upon plants which are of so firm a texture, that they will not easily yield forth their useful parts. In these the ingredients are to be boiled in the water; as, in the others, the boiling water was to be poured over them. In general, leaves, flowers, and entire plants, whether fresh or dried, are used in infusions; the roots and barks in decoctions.

An earthen pipkin, with a close cover, is the best vessel for preparing these; for many of those medicines which are little suspected of it, will take a tincture from the metal; and it would be as improper to boil them in a copper pan, (as it is too common a custom,) as to beat the herbs and roots in a metal mortar.

Fresh roots are used in decoction, as well as those which are dried; and the barks and other ingredients in like manner. When the fresh are used, the roots are to be cut into thin slices, and the barks and woods should be shaved down; as to the leaves and entire plants, they need be cut but slightly. When dry ingredients are used, the roots and barks are best pounded to pieces; and as to the herbs and flowers, little is to be done to them, and in general, they are best added toward the end of the decoction.

It is always best to let the ingredients of a decoction stand in the water cold for twelve hours, before it is set on the fire, and then it should be heated gradually, and afterwards kept boiling gently as long as is necessary: and this is to be proportioned to the nature of the ingredients. Generally a quarter of an hour is sufficient, sometimes much longer is necessary. They are then to be strained off while they are hot, pressing them hard, and the liquor set by to cool: when they are thoroughly cold, they are to be poured off clear from the settlement, for they always become clear as they cool, and sweetened with a little sugar. Frequently also, it is proper to add to them a little white wine, as to the infusions.

Concerning Distilled Waters, and Other Preparations to be Kept in the House.

That spirit is best which is called molasses spirit; it is to be bought at a small price at the distillers; and as to the sugar, the most ordinary loaf kind will do for most purposes; where other is necessary, it will be particularly named.

Few families are without an alembic or still; and that will be of material service. With that instrument the simple waters are to be made, with no expense beside the fire; and it will be proper to keep those of the following ingredients.

Mint-water, peppermint-water, and pennyroyal-water, are to be made of the dry herbs. Three pounds of each is to be put into the still, with four gallons of water, and two gallons is to be distilled off. Milk-water is to be made thus: a pound and half of spear-mint, a pound of rue, half a pound of Roman wormwood, and half a pound of angelica leaves, are to be put into the still with five gallons of water, and three gallons are to be distilled off. Common mint-water is good in sicknesses of the stomach, peppermint-water in colics, and pennyroyal to promote the menses. Milk-water is good in fevers, and to make juleps. It used to be made with milk, but that answers no purpose. Only one simple water more need be kept, and that for colics; it is best made of Jamaica pepper: a pound of Jamaica pepper is to be put into a still over night, with three gallons of water; and the next morning two gallons of water distilled off.

It has been customary to keep a great many simple waters, but these are all that are necessary or proper. The other herbs

263

are better to be given in infusion and decoction.

As for cordial waters, they are made as the others, only with the addition of spirit. It may be proper to keep the following; and no more are necessary.

1. Cinnamon-water; which is made by putting into the still a pound of cinnamon, a gallon of spirit, and a gallon of water, and the next day distilling off a gallon. This is good in sickness of the stomach, and is a fine cordial.

2. Spirituous milk-water; made from a pound of spearmint, half a pound of angelica, and a quarter of a pound of Roman wormwood, all green. To these is to be put a gallon of spirit, and a gallon of water, and a gallon to be distilled off; to which is to be added a pint of vinegar: this is good to promote sweat, and is used instead of treacle-water, being better.

3. Strong pennyroyal-water; which is used instead of hysteric water in all hysteric cases, and to promote the menses, is made of a pound and half of dry pennyroyal, a gallon of spirit, and six quarts of water, drawing off a gallon.

4. Aniseed-water; which is good in the colic, and is made with a pound of aniseed, a pound of angelica seed, and two gallons of spirit, with one gallon of water, distilling off two gallons. No more of these are necessary: but it may be acceptable to add the making of lavender water, spirit of lavender, and Hungary water, which are preparations of the same kind, and very easy.

Lavender-water is made from a pound of fresh lavender flowers, and a gallon of molasses spirit, with two quarts of water; five pints are to be distilled off. Hungary-water is made of a pound and half of rosemary tops with the flowers, a gallon of spirit, and a gallon of water, distilling off five pints: and to make the spirit of lavender, or palsy drops, mix three pints of lavender-water, and one pint of Hungary-water, and add to this half an ounce of cinnamon, the same quantity of nutmegs, and three drachms of red saunders-wood: these are to stand together till the spirit is well coloured.

This is all the family practitioner will need with distilling: a short account, but sufficient.

As for tinctures, which are a great article with the apothecary and chemist, making a great show, and really very useful; I would have several of them kept, and they are as easily made as the waters, nay, more easily. Molasses spirit is all that is necessary for this purpose.

It would be well to keep tinctures of all roots and barks which are recommended to be dried in the course of this work, for a tincture will contain more or less of the virtue of every one of these, and be often convenient, where the powder or decoction could not be given. It is needless to enumerate these, and one rule of making serves for them all: two ounces of the ingredient is to be cut into thin slices, or bruised in a mortar, and put into a quart of spirit; it is to stand a fortnight in a place a little warm, and be often shook; at the end of this time, it is to be taken out, strained off, and made to pass through a funnel, lined with whitish brown paper, and put up with the name of the ingredient.

To these tinctures of roots, barks, and seeds, it would be well to add a few made of foreign ingredients. As,

1. The bitter tincture for the stomach, is made of two ounces of gentian, an ounce of dried orange peel, and half an ounce of cardamom seeds, and a quart of spirit: or it may be made in white wine, allowing two quarts.
2. Tincture of castor, good in hysteric complaints; and made with two ounces of castor and a quart of spirit.
3. Tincture of bark, which will cure those who will not

take the powder; made of four ounces of bark, and a quart of spirit.

4. Tincture of soot, for fits; made with two ounces of wood-soot, one ounce of assafoetida, and a quart of spirit.

5. Tincture of steel, for the stoppage of the menses; made of flowers of iron four ounces, and spirit a quart.

6. Tincture of myrrh, good for curing the scurvy in the gums; made of three ounces of myrrh, and a quart of spirit.

7. Tincture of rhubarb; made of two ounces of rhubarb, half an ounce of cardamom seeds, and a quarter of an ounce of saffron, with a quart of spirit.

8. Elixir salutis; made of a pound of stoned raisins, a pound of senna, an ounce and half of carraway seeds, and half an ounce of cardamoms, in a gallon of spirit.

9. Elixir of vitriol; made of six drachms of cinnamon, three drachms of cardamoms, two drachms of long pepper, and the same of ginger; and a quart of spirit: to a pint of this tincture strained clear off, is to be added four ounces of oil of vitriol: this is an excellent stomachic. Lastly, to these it may be well to add the famous Friar's balsam, which is made of three ounces of benjamin, two ounces of strained storax, one ounce of balsam of Tolu, half an ounce of aloes, and a quart of spirit of wine, such as is burnt under lamps. This spirit may be made by putting a gallon of molasses spirit into the still, and drawing off two quarts, and this will be useful for spirit of wine and camphire, which is made by dissolving an ounce of camphire in a quart of the spirit. Lastly, we are to add what is called the asthmatic elixir, made with flower of benjamin and opium, of each a drachm, camphire two scruples, oil of aniseed forty drops, liquorice root half an ounce, honey one ounce, and a quart of spirit. This is a gentle opiate, and is much better in families than the strong laudanum.

As to the tinctures made with white wine instead of spirit, a few are sufficient. Steel wine is made of a quarter of a pound of filings of iron, and half an ounce of mace, and the same quantity of cinnamon, put into two quarts of Rhenish. Hiera picra is made of half a pound of aloes, two ounces of Winter's bark, and five quarts of white wine. The first is a restorative cordial and strengthener: the latter is sufficiently known as a purge. Laudanum is made of two ounces of opium, a drachm of cloves, and a drachm of cinnamon, and a pint of wine. Viper wine is made of two ounces of dried vipers, and two quarts of white wine: and the tincture of ipecacuanha for a vomit, of two ounces of that root, half an ounce of dry orange peel, and a quart of sack. Lastly, what is called elixir proprietatis is made of aloes, myrrh, and saffron, of each an ounce, sal ammoniac six drachms, and salt of tartar eight ounces, in a quart of mountain wine.

These are all the tinctures and wines that need be kept in a family, whose charity is designed to be very extensive; the expense of the whole is a trifle not worth naming, and the trouble scarce any thing. Books are full of directions in particular for every tincture, as if every one were to be made a different way; but the best method is to give a good deal of time, and frequent shaking, and that will stand in the place of heat in most things of this kind: nevertheless, they should stand in a room where a fire is kept while they are making; and those which require heat, that is, those that take a colour most slowly, are to be placed nearest to it.

Easy as these are, they are by far the most difficult part of the task, the rest is as it were nothing. Conserves, syrups, and ointments will be wanting; but in the same manner one direction will serve for the making the whole assortment of each, and the ingredients will be at hand. As to plaisters in general, they do more harm than good. Surgeons at this time make very little use of them; and in the course of this work, many herbs will be named, the bruised leaves of which are better than all the plasters in the world.

Conserves should be made of rue, mint, scurvy-grass, wood-sorrel, and Roman wormwood. As to the four first, the leaves are to be picked off from the stalks, and beaten up with three times the weight of sugar. The tops of the young shoots of the latter are to be cut off, and they are to be beat up in the same manner. In the course of this work, many plants will be named, the green tops of which contain their virtue, these may all be made into conserves in the same manner, or as many of them added to those here named as shall be thought proper.

Conserves of the flowers of rosemary, mallows, archangel, and lavender, are to be made also in the same manner, and of red-rose buds. These last are to be picked from the husk, and the white heels are to be cut off. They are all to be beat up with three times their weight of sugar; and in the same manner may be made conserves of cowslip flowers, and of those of many other plants mentioned in the following pages.

The outer rind of Seville oranges and lemons, are also to be made into conserves in the same manner, beating them first to a pulp, and then adding the sugar; and to these must be added the conserve of hips and sloes, which are to be made in a particular manner. The hips are to be gathered when fully ripe, afterwards set by in a cellar till they grow very soft; then they are to be laid upon the back of a large hair sieve, a dish being put underneath; they are to be broke with the hand or a wooden pestle, and rubbed about till all the soft matter is forced through the hair-cloth, the seeds and skins only remaining. This soft matter is to be weighed, and to be beat up in a mortar with twice its weight of loaf sugar, first powdered.

Sloes are to be gathered when they are moderately ripe, and they are to be set over the fire in water, till they swell and are softened, but not till the skin bursts; they are then to be laid upon a sieve, and the soft matter driven through, as in the other case; and three times the quantity of sugar is to be mixed with this, that it may make a conserve by beating together.

Syrups are to be made of many ingredients: they may be made indeed of any infusion, with sugar added to it in a due quantity; and the way to add this, so that the syrups shall keep and not candy, is to proportion the sugar to the liquor very exactly. One rule will serve for all this matter, and save a great deal of repetition. The liquor, of which a syrup is to be made, may be the juice of some herb or fruit, or a decoction, or an infusion; whichever it be, let it stand till quite clear; then, to every wine pint of it, add a pound and three quarters of loaf sugar, first beat to powder; put the sugar and the liquor together into an earthen pan that will go into a large saucepan; put water in the saucepan, and set it over the fire. Let the pan stand in it till the sugar is perfectly melted, scumming it all the time; then, as soon as it is cold, it may be put up for use, and will keep all the year round.

This being set down as the general method of making the liquor into a syrup, the rest of the descriptions of them will be easy. They are to be made in this manner: For syrup of cloves, weigh three pounds of clove July flowers picked from the husks, and with the white heels cut off; pour upon them five pints of boiling water. Let them stand all night, and in the morning pour off the clear liquor, and make it into a syrup, as directed above: in the same manner are to be made the syrups of violets and red poppies: but less of the violet flowers will do, and more of the poppies may be added: thus, also, are to be made the syrups of damask roses, peach-blossoms, cowslip-flowers, and many others which will be recommended for that purpose in this book.

Syrup of buckthorn is to be made by boiling the juice

down to half its quantity, with a little cinnamon, ginger, and nutmeg, and then adding the sugar.

The syrups of lemon-juice, mulberries, and the like, are to be made with a pound and half of sugar to every pint of the clear juice, which is to be melted, as in the former manner.

Syrup of garlic, leeks, orange-peel, lemon-peel, mint, and many other things, are to be made of strong infusions of those ingredients, made as before directed, with the first-mentioned quantity of sugar added to them, when they have stood to settle.

Syrup of marshmallows, and of poppy heads, and some others, are to be made in the same manner with the strongest decoctions that can possibly be made from those ingredients, with the same quantity of sugar as is first mentioned.

Syrup of balsam is made by boiling a quarter of a pound of balsam of Tolu, in a pint and half of water, in a close vessel, and then making the water into a syrup, with the usual quantity of sugar: and thus may be made syrups of any of the balsams.

Syrup of saffron is made of a strong tincture of saffron in wine. An ounce of saffron being put to a pint of mountain, and this, when strained off, is to be made into a syrup with the usual quantity of sugar.

At one time it was a custom to keep a quantity of syrups of a particular kind under the name of honeys. They were made with honey instead of sugar, and some of them, which had vinegar in the composition, were called oxymels. A few of the first kind, and very few, are worth keeping, and two or three of the latter, for they have very particular virtues. The way of making them is much the same with that of making syrups; but, to be exact, it may be proper just to give some instances of it.

Honey of roses is the most useful, and it is to be made of an infusion of the flowers and honey in this manner. Cut the white heels from some red-rose buds, and lay them to dry in a place where there is a draught of air; when they are dried, put half a pound of them into a stone jar, and pour on them three pints of boiling water; stir them well, and let them stand twelve hours; then press off the liquor, and when it has settled, add to it five pounds of honey, boil it well, and when it is of the consistence of a thick syrup, put it by for use. It is good against sore mouths, and on many other occasions. In the same manner may be made the honey of any flower; or with the juice of any plant thus mixed with honey, and boiled down, may be made what is called the honey of that plant. As to the oxymels, they are also made in a very uniform manner. The following are so useful, that it will be proper always to keep them in readiness.

For oxymel of garlic, put half a pint of vinegar into an earthen pipkin, boil it in a quarter of an ounce of carraway seeds, and the same quantity of sweet fennel seeds, at last add an ounce and half of fresh garlic root sliced thin; let it boil a minute or two longer, then cover it up to stand till cold, then press out the liquor, and add ten ounces of honey, and boil it to a consistence.

For vinegar of squills, put into a pint of vinegar three ounces of dried squills; let it stand two days in a gentle heat, then press out the vinegar, and when it has stood to settle, add a pound and a half of honey, and boil it to a consistence. Both these are excellent in asthmas.

To these also should be added, the common simple oxymel, which is made of a pint of vinegar, and two pounds of honey, boiled together to the consistence of a syrup.

Finally, as to ointments, nothing can be so easy as the making them of the common herbs; and the expense is only so much hog's-lard. The lard is to be melted, and the fresh-gathered leaves of the herb are to be chopped to pieces, and thrown into it: they are to be boiled till the leaves begin to feel crisp, and then the lard is to be strained off. It will be green, and will have the virtues of the herb, and must be called ointment of such an herb. To these I shall take the opportunity of adding the way to make two or three more, which, though not the produce of English herbs, are very useful, and no family should be without them.

1. The white ointment, called unguentum: this is made by melting together four ounces of white wax, and three ounces of spermaceti, in a pint of salad oil, and adding, if it be desired, three ounces of ceness, and a drachm and half of camphire; but it is better, for all common purposes, without these.

2. Yellow basilicon; which is made by melting together yellow wax, resin, and burgundy pitch, of each half a pound, in a pint of oil of olives, and adding three ounces of turpentine.

3. Black basilicon; which is made by melting together, in a pint of olive oil, yellow wax, resin, and pitch, of each nine ounces.

4. The mercurial ointment, which is thus made: rub together, in an iron mortar, a pound of quicksilver, and an ounce of turpentine; when they are well mixed, add four pounds of hog's-lard melted, and mix all thoroughly together. The ointment of tutty is prepared with levigated tutty, and as much viper's fat as will make it into a soft ointment: these are only to be mixed together upon a marble, by working them with a thin knife. This is for disorders of the eyes; the foregoing for the itch, and many other complaints, but it must be used cautiously. And those which were before named, for old sores.

Of the same nature with the ointments, are, in some degree, the oils made by infusion of herbs and flowers in common oil. These are also very easily prepared, and an instance or two will serve to explain the making of them all. The most regarded among these is the oil of St. John's-wort, and that is thus made: pick clean a quarter of a pound of the flowers of Common St. John's-wort, pour upon them a quart of olive-oil, and let them stand together till the oil is of a reddish colour. Oil of elder is made of a pound of elder flowers, which are to be put into a quart of olive oil, and boiled till they are crisp, and the oil is to be then strained off.

5. What is called the green oil, is thus made: bruise in a marble mortar three ounces of green camomile, with the same quantity of bay leaves, sea-wormwood, rue, and sweet-marjoram; then boil them in a quart of oil of olives, till they are a little crisp. The oil is then to be poured off, and when cold, put up for use.

These oils are used to rub the limbs when there is pain and swellings; their virtues will be found at large, under the several herbs which are the principal ingredients: and after one or other of these methods, may be made the oil by infusion, or by boiling of any plant, or of any number of plants, of like virtue.

Lastly, though herbs are now left out of the composition of plasters, even the melilot being now made without the herb from which it was first named, it may be proper to add the way of preparing a few that are most useful, and ought to be kept in families.

1. The common plaster is thus made; boil together a gallon of oil, five pounds of powdered litharge, and a quart and four ounces of water. When the water is boiled away, the rest will be united into a plaster, but it must be stirred all the time: this

273

used to be called diachylon. To make diachylon with the gums, add to a pound of the last described, two ounces of galbanum, and an ounce of common turpentine, and the same quantity of frankincense. Melt them all together, the gums first, and then add the plaster.

2. For a strengthening plaster; melt two pounds of the common plaster, and add to it half a pound of frankincense, and three ounces of dragon's blood.

3. For a drawing plaster; melt together yellow wax and yellow resin, of each three pounds, and a pound of mutton suet. This is used, instead of the old melilot plaster, to dress blisters; and the blister plaster itself is made of it, only by adding half a pint of vinegar, and a pound of Spanish flies in powder, to two pounds of it, just as it begins to cool from melting. The quicksilver plaster is thus made; rub three ounces of quicksilver, with a drachm of balsam of sulphur, till it no longer appears in globules, then pour in a pound of the common plaster melted, and mix them well together.

A few recipes for making waters without distillation, are added, which being cheap and very serviceable, ought not to be omitted.

1. Lime-water; this is made by pouring gradually six quarts of water upon a pound of quick lime; when it has stood to be clear, it must be poured off. If a pound of lignum-vitae wood, an ounce of liquorice root, and half an ounce of sassafras bark, be added to three quarts of lime-water, it is called compound lime-water, and is excellent in foulnesses of the blood.

2. The blue eye-water; this is made by putting a drachm of sal ammoniac into a pint of lime-water, and letting it stand in a brass vessel, till it is of a sky-blue colour.

274

3. Alum-water is made by boiling half an ounce of white vitriol, and the same quantity of alum, in a quart of water, till they are dissolved.

Thus have we described all the drugs and compositions that need be kept for family use, or to relieve the neighbouring poor in their greatest of all distresses, that of sickness.

Concerning the Best Methods of Putting Medicines Together for Present Taking.

In the first place, although these several forms of syrups, conserves, and the like, have been named, as what will be sometimes necessary; the great practice in the country will lie in the infusions and decoctions of the fresh plants and roots.

The strength of these infusions and decoctions is to be proportioned to the taste: for as they are made to be swallowed in quantities, if they be made so strong as to be very disagreeable, that end will be defeated: they may be rendered more pleasant by sweetening them with sugar, about an ounce of which is to be allowed to a quart; and occasionally a little white wine, or a small quantity of some of the cordial waters, may be added to them. The dose of either decoction or infusion, will be in general about half a pint, except where they are intended to purge or vomit; there they must be more carefully and exactly proportioned to the strength, than can be told in this general manner.

Of the simple water, about a quarter of a pint is a dose; and of the cordial waters, less than half that quantity. These may be occasionally given alone; but they are mostly intended for mixing with other ingredients.

The tinctures are to be given in drops, from ten to an hundred, according to their strength and nature; but to name a general dose, it is about five and twenty drops. These, however, will be also more serviceable in mixtures, than singly. Of the purging tinctures in wine, and the elixir salutis, three, four, or more spoonfuls, is the dose.

It would be well to keep tinctures of many of the roots recommended in nervous cases, as cordials, astringents, and of many other kinds; and also to keep powders of these roots in readiness: and thus the common forms of medicines, as sent from apothecaries, will be very easy.

For julep, six ounces of one of the simple waters, two ounces of one of the compound waters, or those made with spirit, two drachms of a syrup, and fifty drops of a tincture, make a very agreeable one. Thus, for an hysteric julep, let the simple water be pennyroyal, the strong water the strong pennyroyal, the syrup that of saffron, and the tincture of castor; and it is a very pleasant julep: and so of all the rest. If a pearl cordial be desired, it is only mixing the simple and strong waters without syrup or tincture, and adding two drachms of sugar, and half a drachm of levigated oyster-shells. —The apothecaries will not be pleased with thus disclosing the mysteries of their profession; but the public good is of more consequence than their pleasure.

Draughts are only little juleps, with more powerful ingredients added to them. An ounce and half of a simple water, three drachms of a strong water, one drachm of a syrup, and forty drops of a tincture, make a draught; but to these may be added a simple of some power, to increase the virtue. What waters, tinctures, syrups, or powders, shall be used, will be determined from the case itself.

276

Boluses are made with these powders in a certain dose. A scruple, or half a drachm, is made into a sort of paste with syrup. The common custom is to cover it with a little leaf-gold, but this is better let alone: some use leaf-brass, which is abominable.

Electuaries are to be made of powders, conserves, and syrups; they differ from boluses in this, as well as in the size, that the dose is smaller, although the piece taken be as large; which is owing to the conserve, that having in general little virtue in comparison of the other ingredients. This is the form most convenient for medicines that are to be taken for a continuance of time, and the dose of which needs not be so very punctually regarded.

Thus, for an electuary against an habitual looseness, when it exceeds the proper bounds; mix together an ounce of conserve of red roses, and six drachms of syrup of cloves; add to these, two drachms of powdered bistort root, one drachm of powdered tormentil, and half a drachm of toasted rhubarb. This makes an electuary, a piece of which, of the bigness of a nutmeg, taken once in two days, will check the abundance of stools, without stopping the customary looseness entirely: it will also be a pleasant medicine. If a draught of tincture of roses be taken after this, it will increase the power.

In this manner any person may supply the place of the apothecary, to those who could not afford such assistance: and experience is so good a guide, that they will be able in most cases to save the expense of the doctor also; with very little danger of doing harm. The Galenical physic, perhaps, will be found effectual in many more cases, by those who stick to it solely, than they are aware who do not use it: as to the mischief of medicine, that is almost entirely chemical. It would be idle to say that chemical medicines do not do great good; but they require to be in skilful hands: when the ignorant employ them, death is more likely to be the consequence, than the relief from the disorder any other way.

Concerning the Virtues of Plants which have not yet been tried.

The number of English plants, whose virtues are ascertained, scarcely exceeds one thousand, while the catalogue of those which are natives of our own country, as published by Mr. Ray, amounts to many thousands: great numbers therefore remain yet untried, and present an ample field for our researches.

To what purpose can a man devote the hours of his leisure better, than to the discovering, among the number of the unregarded, virtues which may farther supply the catalogue of our own remedies, and make the roots and seeds brought from remote countries less necessary? What encouragement to the attempt, that there are such multitude of objects for the trial! and that the discovering but one remedy among them all, for a disease we knew not how so well to cure before, is a source of more true honour, than can be derived from all the useless knowledge in the world.

If any suppose the trial dangerous, they mislead themselves; and to encourage so laudable an undertaking, I shall observe how little is the hazard, and how considerable the advantages, from what we know already.

If a man were to be turned loose upon an island where no person had set foot before, he might dread to taste of any plant he saw, because he might not know but every one he saw was fatal and supposing him to have got over this fear, the ignorance of the virtues of all would keep him backward: but this is not at all the case with him, who shall at this time set about inquiring into the virtues of plants in England. The poisonous plants, native of our soil, are hardly a dozen, and these are charactered even to the eye, by something singular or dismal in the aspect. They are well known, and he has nothing to do but to avoid them. For the rest, he has so many, whose uses and qualities are already perfectly known, that he has a great foundation to go upon in the search, because he can compare those he does not know with them. Their tastes will go a great way toward informing him: but this is not all, their very outward figures will direct him; for in general those plants which agree in the external aspect, agree likewise in their virtues.

To give an instance in the marshmallow. It is known to work by urine, and to be good against the gravel. We will suppose no more known concerning this kind. A person desirous of extending this useful knowledge, finds that by the taste of the root, which is insipid, and its mucilaginous quality, he might have guessed this to be its virtue, from what he before knew of medicine. The next plant he meets, we will suppose is the common mallow, and afterwards the little white-flowered mallow, which lies upon the ground; he tastes the roots of these, and he finds they are like the other: he will therefore guess that they have the same virtues, and upon trial he will find it is so.

But this is not all: if he had examined the flower of the marshmallow, in what manner it was constructed, and how the little threads grew within it, he would have found that the flowers of these other two mallows were, in all respects, like those of the other; and farther, he would have found, that the seeds of these two kinds were in the same manner disposed in circular bodies: from this he might, without tasting their roots, have been led to guess that their virtues were the same: or, having guessed so much from this, he might have been thence led to taste them, and by that have been confirmed in it: but he might be carried farther; he would find the same sort of round clusters of seeds in the hollyoak in his garden; and upon examining the single flowers, he would see they were also alike: and hence he would discover that it was of this kind; and he would rightly judge that the holly-oak also possessed the same virtues.

There is this great use in examining other plants which have the same sort of flowers and fruits with those which we know to have virtues, that we may in this way discover plants at home, to supply the place of those we have from other countries. It is certain the sun in warmer climates does ripen the juices of vegetables faster than in ours, but yet we find the plants of the same kind, from whatever part of the world they come, to possess nearly the same kind of virtues; generally indeed they are the same, only differing in degree. Thus all the mallows of Spain and Italy, to bring the trial to the before-named instance, possess the same virtues with the marshmallow, mallow, and hollyoak of England; and the case is the same with those which are truly mallows of the East and West Indies; though this does not hold good with respect to some of the plants of those countries which have been brought hither under that name. Thus the senega rattlesnake root, which was once much in use amongst us, has been discovered to belong to a kind of milkwort, or polygala. The roots of the common milkwort of our pastures being tried, have been found to possess the same virtues, though in a less degree. This plant would not have been regarded, if the other had not been found to be of the same kind; but to that we owe the knowledge of its virtues.

There is this great reason for seeking in our own climate, plants of the same nature, form, and kind, with those which in other countries afford us remedies — that they are generally of the same kind, and maybe fitter for our constitutions; for as it has been before observed, the productions of each respective country, are always best suited to supply the wants of its inhabitants both for food and medicine: and it is certain, that as the sun ripens the juices of plants in hotter countries to more virtue than with us, so it makes men's constitutions more able to bear their effects.

The Chinese will swallow such doses as would poison one of us. This we know in many instances, and it ought to encourage us in the present research: because, if the same doses which agree with them are too much for us, we may also find that other medicines of our own growth, and of the same kind of virtues, though in a less degree, may also be found to agree better with our constitutions. Therefore, notwithstanding that it may be necessary in some cases, and convenient in many, for us to have drugs from abroad, yet in general it will be better; for us to be cured by those herbs we may find at home; and they will be found upon trial more sufficient for that purpose than we at present imagine. The means are at hand, but we have made very little use of them, proportioned to their number and their value.

The observation already made, that the external form of plants may very well give the hint for a conjecture about their virtues, is much more general than might be imagined. Almost all the plants of the same kinds are of the same virtues. But that is not all; for, in general, those of the same class possess the same qualities, though different in degree: and this is a prodigious help to him who shall set out upon the generous and useful plan of adding to the number of the useful plants. It is also singular, that what might appear objections in this case, being brought to the trial, will often be found confirmations of the truth there is in the observation.

Thus, suppose a man, observing that lettuce is eatable, should inquire into all the plants like lettuce, which are those that have flowers composed of many parts, and have the seeds winged with a white downy matter, to find whether they were eatable; let us examine how he would succeed. The plants of this class native of England, are, the sowthistle, the hawkweeds, the dandelions, goats-beards, succory, and endive, all eatables. The hawkweeds are less agreeable in the taste, but wholesome; and as to the wild lettuces, those who would bring the opiate quality of the principal of them as an objection, strengthen the observation, for the garden lettuce also has an opiate quality. This wild one possesses it in a greater degree, but still in such a degree, that it is an excellent medicine, not at all dangerous. Its bitter taste would prevent people's eating it, for it is disagreeable; but its virtues are the same with those of lettuce, only greater. There are some kinds of hawkweed also, which have a bitter milky juice, altogether like that of this lettuce; and they also have the same opiate quality.

This general observation may be carried a great deal farther. In general, the seeds of umbelliferous plants, that is, those which have little flowers in rounded clusters, each succeeded by two seeds, are good against colics; those of carraway, anise, cummin, coriander, and all of that kind, are produced by plants of this figure. In the same manner the verticillate plants, as they are called, that is, those which have the flowers surrounding the stalks, as in mint and thyme, are of a warm nature; and however they differ in degree and circumstance, they have the same general virtues. Farther, such plants as are insipid to the taste and smell, have generally little virtues; and, on the contrary, those which have the most fragrant smell and sharpest taste, have the greatest virtues, of whatever kind.

In general also, those plants which have a strong but an agreeable taste, are most worthy to be examined with respect to their virtues; for they are generally the most valuable: and, on the contrary, when a very strong taste is also a very disagreeable one; or, in the same manner, when the strong smell of a plant has also something heavy, disagreeable, and overpowering in it; there is mischief in the herb, rather than any useful quality. The poisonous plants of this country are very few; but they are for the most part characterized after this manner so that they are known as it were at sight, or by the first offer of a trial.

BIBLIOGRAPHY

For the benefit of the reader, the author herein gives a list of the origins of most of the data used in this book.

This is a most varied, unusual and imposing compilation. It consists of references, tomes, abstracts, volumes, treatises, manuscripts, works, books and booklets pertaining to herbs and herbalism.

Let he who dares challenge the validity of the authorities cited.

AUTHOR (Or Compiler)	WORK	ORIGIN	DATE Approx.
Moses	Bible	Hebrew	4004 B.C.
Enlil-Bani, King of Isin	Tablets	Egyptian	2201 B.C.
Ebers	Papyrus	Egyptian	2000 B.C.
Solomon	Bible	Hebrew	1000 B.C.
Homer	Iliad & Odyssey	Greek	700 B.C.
Daniel	Bible	Hebrew	600 B.C.
Hippocrates	Aphorisms & The Airs	Greek	460-370 B.C.
Aristotle	Organum	Greek	384-322 B.C.
Theophrastus	History of Plants	Greek	372-287 B.C.
Pliny	Naturales Historia	Roman	23-79 A.D.
Dioscorides	"De Materia Medica"	Greek	40-100 A.D.
Unknown	Pseudo-Apuleius		Unknown
Galen	Various Treatises	Greek	130-200 A.D.
Sammonicus (Serenus)	Praecepta de Medicina	Roman	212 A.D.
Emperor Charlemagne	Garden of Herbs	French	742-814 A.D.
Unknown	The Herbarius zu Teutsch Herbarium vivae escones de Historia stirpium	German	1485

AUTHOR	WORK	ORIGIN	DATE
Unknown	Hortus sanitatis		1491
Paracelsus	114 Experiments & Cures and Doctrine of Signatures	Swiss	1493-1541
Bartholomew	Herbal	English	1495
Banckes	Herbal		1525
Brunfels, Otto		German	1530
Della Porta, G.B.	Magia Naturalis, Doctrine of Signatures	Italian	1538-1615
Fuchs, Leonhard	Unknown		1542
Mattioli	Commentaries on the Six Books of Dioscorides	Italian	1544
Gerard, John	The Herbal, General History of Plants	English	1545-1612
Turner, Wm.	Libellus de re Herbaria	English	1551-1568
Parkinson, John	Paradisus Terrestris Theatrum Botanicum	English	1567-1629
Coles, Wm.	The Art of Simpling	English	1650
Culpeper, Nicholas	The Complete Herbal and English Physician	English	1616-1654
Salmon, Wm., M.D.	History of Plants	English	1710
Miller, Joseph	Botanicum Officinale	English	1722
Hill, John	British Herbal	English	1756
Brook, Richard	A New Family Herbal		Prior to 1800
Green, Thos.	Universal Herbal		18..
Thornton, J.T., M.D.	A New Family Herbal		1810
Buchan, Wm.	Domestic Medicine		Prior to 1839
Barton, B.H. and Castle, Thos.	The Medicinal Plants of Great Britain		1845
Robinson, Matt, M.D.	The New Family Herbal		Prior to 1910
Arber, Agnes	Herbals: Their Origin and Evolution		
Bailey, Liberty Hyde	The Standard Cyclopedia of Horticulture		
Bethel, May	The Healing Power of Herbs		
Brandt, Johanna	The Grape Cure		
Colin, Jane	Herbs and Spices		
Fox, Wm., M.D.	Family Botanic Guide		
Freeman, Margaret	Herbs for the Medieval Household		

AUTHOR	WORK	ORIGIN	DATE
Geuter, Maria	Herbs in Nutrition		
Greyson	A Herbal of Sorts		
Grieve, M.	A Modern Herbal		
Harper-Shrove, F.	Medicinal Herbs		
Harris, B.C., Ph.G.R.P.	Kitchen Medicines		
James, Claudia V.	Herbs & The Fountain of Youth		
Krutch, Jos. Wood	Herbal		
Leyel, Mrs. C.F.	Herbal Delights, Elixirs of Life, Herbs for the Heart, Compassionate Herbs, Hearts-Ease, Green Medicine,Cinquefoil		
Lingard, W. Burns, F.N.I.M.H.	Herbal Prescriptions		
Loewenfeld, Claire	Herbal Gardening		
Meyer, Jos. E.	The Herbalist		
Paxton, Sir Jos.	Botanical Dictionary		
Porter, Frank W.	Miracle Workers		
Quelch, Mary Thorne	The Herb Garden, Herbal Remedies, and Herbs for Daily Use		
Rhode, Eleanor	The Old English Herbal		
Seymour, E.D.	The New Garden Encyclopedia		
de Sounin, Leonie	Magic in Herbs		
Steinmetz, E.F.	Materia Medica Vegetablis		
Taylor, Norman	Encyclopedia of Gardening		
Webster, Helen Noyes	Herbs		
Wren, R.C., F.L.S.	New Encyclopedia of Botanical Drugs and Preparations		
Yemm, J.R.	The Medical Herbalist		
	Herbalist Hand Book		
	Universal Botanic Guide		
	Encyclopedia Britannica		
	Columbia Encyclopedia		
	The Royal Horticultural Society Dictionary of Gardening		

287

INDEX OF COMMON NAMES

291

INDEX OF BOTANICAL NAMES

295

Pedalium murex, 76
Petasites vulgaris, 10
Peumus boldus, 71
Phytolacca decandra, 67
Pilocarpus microphyllus, 44
Pinus mugo, 87
Pinus sylvestris, 87
Piper methysticum, 103
Piper nigrum, 35
Pistacia lentiscus, 60
Plantago major, 20
Plantago psyllium, 80
Podophyllum peltatum, 33,190
Polemonium reptans, 78
Polygonatum multiflorum, 24
Polygonum bistorta, 119
Polygonum hydropiper, 157
Polymnia uvedalia, 89
Polyporus fomentarius, 79
Pomaderris elliptica, 103
Populus candicans, 29
Populus tremuloides, 134
Portulaca oleracea, 39
Potentilla anserina, 62
Potentilla reptans, 132
Potentilla tormentilla, 117
Primula vulgaris, 174
Prunella vulgaris, 81
Prunus persica, 64
Punica granatum, 91

Quercus infectoria, 156

Ranunculus ficaria, 114
Rhamnus purshiana, 115
Rheum palmatum, 150

Rhus toxicodendron, 10
Ribes nigrum, 156
Ricinus communis, 98
Rosa canina, 95
Rosmarinus officinalis, 119
Rubus idaeus, 130
Rubus villosus, 44
Rumex acetosa, 41
Rumex aquaticus, 68
Rumex crispus, 191
Ruscus aculeatus, 83
Ruta graveolens, 38,152,191

Salix alba, 45
Salix discolor, 137
Salvia officinalis, 115
Salvia sclarea, 56
Sanicula europaea, 28
Sarracenia purpurea, 140
Satureia hortensis, 138
Schoenocaulon officinale, 170
Scolopendrium vulgare, 89
Scutellaria laterifolia, 72
Sedum acre, 190
Senecio aureus, 150
Senecio maritimus, 27
Serenoa serrulata, 11
Sesamum indicum, 28
Silphium perfoliatum, 143
Simaba cedron, 8
Sisymbrium officinale, 72
Smilax ornata, 152
Solidago virgaurea, 129
Sorghum vulgare, 167
Spiraea ulmaria, 29
Stachys betonica, 47,191

INDEX OF AILMENTS
AND USES

303